INTERMITTENT FASTING: BEGINNER'S GUIDE TO WEIGHT LOSS FOR MEN AND WOMEN OVER 50

LOVE YOURSELF AGAIN! LOSE WEIGHT AND KEEP IT OFF, GET FIT AND FEEL HEALTHY, PLUS BONUS RECIPES AND A 21-DAY MEAL PLAN

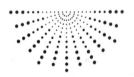

KOOROSH NAGHSHINEH

SELF-PUBLISHED

TABLE OF CONTENTS

About this Book vii

Part I

THE WHAT AND HOW OF INTERMITTENT
FASTING

Introduction 3

1. INTERMITTENT FASTING DEFINED 5
History of Intermittent Fasting 7
When IF Became Popular 9
Kathy's Journey 10
Things to Remember 10

2. SCIENCE DOESN'T LIE 12
What the Mice Say 12
Studies on Humans 13
Things to Remember 14

3. BENEFITS FOR PEOPLE OVER 50 (AND POSSIBLE
RISKS) 16
What We Are All Here For: Weight Loss 16
Other Benefits 20
Potential Risks 22
Mark's Journey 23
Things to Remember 24

4. DIFFERENT TYPES OF IF, YOU'VE GOT OPTIONS 25
Restricted Eating Windows 25
Koorosh's Journey 33
Things to Remember 33

5. TIPS FOR GETTING STARTED 36
Utilize Your Sleeping Hours 36
Plan Ahead 36
Don't Stress—Listen to Your Body 38
Stay Busy 38
Track Your Progress 39

When to Exercise 41

Kathleen's Journey 42

Things to Remember 43

6. YOU ARE WHAT YOU EAT SO CHOOSE CLEAN
EATING 44

Avocado 49

Fish and Seafood 50

Cruciferous Vegetables 51

Potatoes (They Get a Bad Rap!) 51

Beans, Beans, the Magical Fruit 52

Eggs 53

Whole Grains 53

Berries 54

Nuts 55

George's Journey 56

Things to Remember 57

7. MISTAKES AND HOW TO AVOID THEM 58

Stay Focused 58

Be Disciplined 59

Eat the Right Foods 60

Ease Into It 61

Choose the Right Plan 61

Susan's Journey 62

Things to Remember 62

8. HOW TO BREAK YOUR FAST 64

Low-Carb, High-Fat 64

Fruits 65

Bone Broth 65

Apple Cider Vinegar 65

Protein 66

Koorosh's Journey 66

Things to Remember 67

9. CONCLUSIONS 68

Acknowledgments 71

Glossary 73

References 75

Part II
BONUS RECIPES AND MEAL PLAN

10. BREAKFAST RECIPES 95
Protein Berry and Carrot Smoothie 96
Strawberry Yogurt Smoothie 97
Cottage Cheese & Applesauce 98
Scrambled Eggs with Spinach and Cheese 99
Peanut Butter Banana English Muffin 100
Keto Breakfast Tacos 101
Spinach and Sausage Breakfast Muffin 103
Kale and Egg Cups 105
Oatmeal and Apples 107
Avocado and Egg Toast 108

11. LUNCH RECIPES 109
Turkey Salad 109
Chicken Lettuce Wraps 111
Spinach, Lemon, and Shrimp Salad 112
Chicken, Spinach, and Strawberry Salad 113
Flank Steak and Tomatoes 114
BBQ Chicken Salad 116
Cheesy Burger Stuffed Portobellos 118
Paleo Avocado Chicken Salad 120
Paleo Avocado Tuna Salad 121
Mexican Quinoa 122

12. DINNER RECIPES 124
Maple Glazed Chicken 125
Philly Cheesesteak Stuffed Halved Peppers 127
Spinach and Mushroom Smothered Grilled Chicken 129
Baked Chicken with Spinach, Pears and Blue Cheese 131
Lemon Grilled Chicken Breast 133
Grilled Salmon with Dill Butter 134
Chicken and Broccoli 136
Cheesy Chicken and Spinach 138
Bacon and Brussels Sprouts Gratin 139
Balsamic Red Wine Glazed Filet Mignon 141
Lemon Steamed Broccoli 142

13. SNACK IDEAS 143
    Ants on a Log 144
    Apples and Almond Butter 145
    Cinnamon Apple Bites 146
    Apple and Vanilla-Cinnamon Yogurt 147
    Paleo & Keto Chocolate Pudding 148
    Blueberry Muffin 149
    Frozen Yogurt Blueberries 151
    Mango Smoothie 152
    Greek Yogurt with Blueberries, Walnuts & Honey 153
    Rice Cake with Strawberries and Honey 154
    Spinach Avocado Smoothie Bowl 155

14. 21-DAY MEAL PLAN 156
    Sample Meal Plan for 16:8 157
    Meal Plan Template 162

ABOUT THIS BOOK

It was about 3:40 pm one afternoon a few years ago, I was walking back from teaching a class as I fell in step with Fernando. We were both going in the same direction as I was heading to my office. He was one of our best graduate students, had taken many of my classes and aced them. Over time, we had developed a friendship and would chat some times. I asked him where he was going. He said to dinner. I said: "Dinner at this time?" He said: "Yes, I eat now and then don't eat again until breakfast tomorrow. I have been losing weight doing this for the past few months. I am going home to have a large salad for dinner." So I asked more questions and found out this was called Intermittent Fasting (IF, for short).

That was a few years ago. I started researching IF and then began experimenting with it. I found that I slept much better, had more energy, and felt much healthier. My wife and I found that the 16:8 method (will be explained later in this book) worked well for us. I kept notes on the what, the how, and the why of IF as I went along. I joined a couple of Facebook groups for IF and learned more. My weight stabilized at a place that I was very happy with it so I kept doing what I was doing. Today, I still practice IF.

This book is a culmination of all that I have researched and learned. I am not medical doctor or a nutritionist, or a dietitian. I am just sharing with you what worked for me and what I have learned about IF. I want you to learn about this amazing technique, try it over the next few months, and see if it is for you. I advise you to be kind to yourself. Start easy and ramp up as your body adapts to the change in your eating schedule. If you have a medical condition, make sure to talk to your doctor before you try IF. Always remember that you are looking for longterm gains and establishing a lifetime habit, not an overnight success that will disappear in a month or two.

In order to make this process easier for you, I have divided this book in two parts. Part I includes all the material needed to better understand Intermittent Fasting. Part II provides you with some recipes you can try as well as a 21-Day meal plan.

I wish you the best in your IF journey and hope that you achieve the results you are looking for as I have. May your body and spirit always be healthy!

FREE GIFTS FOR THE READER

Thank you for reading *Intermittent Fasting: Beginner's Guide to Weight Loss for Men and Women Over 50*. I hope you will find it insightful, inspiring, and most importantly practical. I hope it helps you lose weight easily and to have a healthy body.

To help you get the best results as fast as possible, I have included the following additional bonus materials at no extra cost to you. These are:

- A weekly meal planner template
- More recipes
- More resources for you to tap into (books, videos, Facebook groups, etc.)

To get your bonuses, please scan this image using your cellphone camera.

Alternatively, you can go to this link:

https://www.betterbalanceforall.com

In both cases, you will be directed to the same website where you will create an account and receive access to this material. My goal is to continue to add useful material to this website to help you succeed in improving your health and balance.

PART I
THE WHAT AND HOW OF
INTERMITTENT FASTING

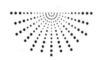

INTRODUCTION

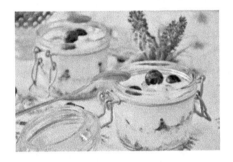

Fasting is like spring cleaning for your body. –Jentezen Franklin

Trying to lose weight can be exhausting. It can feel as though you're on a hamster wheel with no progress in sight. Diets, fads, and guides all end up with the same result, either no weight loss or eventually returning right back where you started. Then, to make weight loss even more difficult, we get older and our bodies change and begin working against us. You see this at times when we reach our 50's and encounter hormonal changes (menopause for women and low testosterone for men). Even those who are nutrition and fitness enthusiasts can struggle with weight gain. Sometimes it feels like your metabolism has slowed down overnight.

But there is something you can do about this and you don't have to endure the added pounds just because you are now over 50. It's time to try a new tactic, a method that is more doable, sustainable, and effective than regular dieting. That is where **intermittent fasting (IF)** comes in. Once you develop a plan that you know you could commit to, the extra weight will fall away (and your clothes begin fitting you like they used to). This is what happened to me and that's why I am writing this book. I want to share IF with you.

Reading this book and developing your plan will give you the same results that it gave me. And, as we will discuss, the benefits of IF go far beyond that of weight loss. Get started on your IF journey today, and start seeing the results you're looking for!

INTERMITTENT FASTING DEFINED

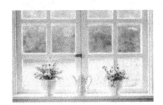

W hen starting on the path of intermittent fasting, it is important to have a firm understanding of what it is, exactly. How did this method of losing weight come about? How does it work? This chapter will give a clear definition of IF and cover the history of how it became the most popular way for people in the United States to lose weight. With a deeper knowledge of the functionality of IF, it is easier to stick with it and be disciplined in the effort to adopt a new weight-loss method.

First and foremost, IF focuses on when to eat rather than what to eat. Eating on a regular schedule and fasting between **eating windows** is the key to effective weight loss and management. Mark Mattson is a neuroscientist at the Johns Hopkins Institute and has studied intermittent fasting for 25 years. According to his research, the human body has evolved to survive, and thrive, for up to several days without food. During hunter/gatherer days, it took a long time and incredible energy to obtain food.

It was only 50 years ago that portions were much smaller, cell phones and laptops were non-existent, and entertainment was more often sought outdoors. It is much easier today to sit and binge-watch our favorite shows while snacking into the night. Unfortunately, this shift in activities and calorie intake has resulted in higher risks of diabetes, obesity, heart disease, and many other illnesses.

Intermittent fasting curbs the risks of modern-day diseases by reducing the eating window during the day. This works to burn fat because there is a **metabolic switch** that takes place after the body has burned all of its sugar stores. Once there isn't any more sugar available, the body begins burning fat instead. This means that for most people that eat on a typical American schedule, three meals a day plus snacks, they are only burning the calories they eat and not burning any stored fat. And unfortunately, if all of the day's consumed calories aren't burned through physical activity, weight gain is the inevitable result.

There are different ways to go about IF but all methods include an eating window. All calories for the day are consumed during the eating window and the remainder of the day is the fasting period. This scheduling of eating windows and fasting windows is also known as **time-restricted eating**. When first starting IF, the goal should be to start with a smaller eating window than is typical for you. There are several schedules that we'll cover in later chapters but starting slow will help sustain IF as a new lifestyle choice.

The term *diet* induces feelings of guilt, failure, and exhaustion of both the physical and mental nature. That is why, for lasting results, one must adopt a different way of living… Or, in this case, eating. IF is not difficult. It is not exhausting (in fact, you will likely feel as though you have more energy throughout the day). And, there is no need to feel guilty because you don't have to restrict what you eat. All of us fast for some time in a day. From the time the last dessert or snack in the evening is consumed until the cup of coffee or breakfast in the morning is the common fasting window for most people. IF starts with just broadening that window a bit. What makes IF so easy is that the bulk of the fasting window is spent sleeping. To start IF, maybe your current fasting window is extended by a mere two hours. An extra hour of fasting at night before bed, and another in the morning before breakfast is a small adjustment that can give big results. The good news is that clear liquids do not contain calories that will break your fast! That means that tea, coffee (forgoing the cream and sugar), and water are always ok.

HISTORY OF INTERMITTENT FASTING

From the evolutionary stand point, fasting has been ingrained in our body's means of processing foods and stored fats. Ancestors that hunted game and gathered vegetation to survive had no means of storing food to eat later. So, it was a way of life to go hours or days fasting involuntarily. With those who could survive the longest without food being those that were also most likely to pass along their genetic code to children, a genetic code was passed from generation to generation. Today, there are several examples of people that have survived long periods of fasting due to the genetic contributions of our hunter/gatherer ancestors. While today, most of us have a choice as to when we eat, fasting is still in our genetic make-up and can benefit us in ways that go beyond weight loss.

There is ancient documentation showing that humans have fasted for as far back as documentation has existed. For the ancient Greeks, fasting was used to improve health and spirituality. Pythagoras (580-500BC) was a philosopher and mathematician that practiced fasting to foster heightened clarity, mental perception, and creativity. Today, scientists have shown that the practices of Pythagoras were valid.

Plato (427-347BC) and Hippocrates (460-357BC) also promoted fasting as one of the first methods of modern medicine. Plato separated medicinal practices into 'true medicine' and 'false medicine' of which fasting was documented to be true and held in the same vein of necessity as air and sun. Hippocrates wrote of eating too richly and thus nourishing disease. His standpoint was that if the body was cleared through fasting then the disease is starved. Funny enough, most of us lose our appetites when we're sick so maybe he was onto something there! The ancient Greeks also used fasting to reduce seizure occurrences in epileptic patients with documented success. Today, we have anticonvulsant drugs so fasting isn't necessary as a treatment course of action.

Other historical mentions of fasting are seen in the Bible and include a 40-day fast before Easter. It is thought that Lent (a Teutonic word translating to *forty days*) was practiced with a festival of Ascension (Purification). It is unknown when the church adopted fasting practices but is common-day, and historically practiced from Clean Monday until Easter.

Modern-day intermittent fasting has relied on the science produced from several studies showing the resulting health benefits. One such study was conducted in 2003 on mice and was led by the head of the National Institute on Aging's neuroscience laboratory, Mark Mattson. The study looked at the levels of glucose and insulin in the blood of mice that were either on restricted caloric intake or intermittently fasting. The IF mice showed higher insulin sensitivity and had a lower incidence of diabetes. Though the mice lived the same durations, the IF mice won out by living healthier in that duration.

Mattson's research went on to show that IF may protect the brain against degenerative diseases that are more common in the later years of life. One of his studies produced results suggesting that the brains of rats exposed to IF were resistant to toxins that damage brain cells leading to stroke, Parkinson's disease, and cognitive decline (a common symptom of Alzheimer's). Mattson has since practiced IF and only eats breakfast and lunch on the weekends, claiming that it helps him be more productive during the week. Note that Mattson does not have a medical degree. He has a Ph.D. in biology and has studied cellular aspects of aging which have resulted in over 700 article publications.

Other results that Mattson has published with his studies on IF with rodents is that it leads to higher levels of brain-derived neurotrophic factor (BDNF) which is a protein that protects neurons from dying under stress. Low levels of this protein have been linked to depression and Alzheimer's disease. Also, fasting seems to increase the rate of autophagy, or the ridding of damaged molecules, which have also been linked to Alzheimer's but also Parkinson's, and some other neurological diseases.

Chicago researchers stated that fasting seemed "to delay the development of the disorders that lead to death." This came after the University of Chicago reported on an experiment involving rats that were dieting daily versus rats that were only fed every other day. The rats exposed to IF lived longer and showed a much lower incidence of disease than the other group.

WHEN IF BECAME POPULAR

In 2012, a documentary was aired called *Eat, Fast, and Live Longer.* It highlighted the benefits of IF and revealed that it was a lifestyle that would lead to weight loss and reduced risk of common aging diseases, such as cancer, Alzheimer's, and heart disease, without restricting the foods we love most. The buzz that was created by the science revealed in this documentary resulted in celebrities giving it a try and increasing the hype even more.

One celebrity that credits her fabulously fit physique to IF is Jennifer Aniston. She admittedly skips breakfast and only consumes clear liquids in the morning. Another is supermodel, Gisele Bundchen, practicing the 5:2 method (we'll cover this more later) by only consuming 500-600 calories two days a week. Others who can personally vouch for the effectiveness include Halle Berry, Scarlett Johansson, and Reese Witherspoon. Another impressively successful celebrity who openly admits that his heightened mental focus and successful weight management are due to his commitment to eating *only* dinner every day of the week is, Jack Dorsey. Jack is the cofounder of both Twitter and Square. He saves his caloric intake for a single-hour window in which he consumes all of the necessary nutrients in a single sitting. This type of fasting is on the more extreme side and should not be attempted initially.

KATHY'S JOURNEY

> "Before I started my IF journey, I was skeptical that it would work for me. After reaching the age of 50, it seemed impossible to lose weight. I had tried diet after diet with nothing but frustration and defeat to show for it. I was convinced that putting on a bit of extra weight was just part of the effects of post-menopausal hormones. Finally, I decided to do some research on IF to find out if it was as effective as everyone was making it out to be. As it turns out, science doesn't lie."
>
> — KATHY, 55 YEARS OLD

THINGS TO REMEMBER

- IF focuses more on when you eat, not as much on what you eat.
- IF consists of eating windows and fasting windows.
- Humans have evolved to go long periods without eating. It's in our DNA.
- IF is easier than people think.
- Both the Ancient Greeks, scientific studies, and current-day role models vouch for the effectiveness of IF.

You're probably convinced that IF is worth a shot at this point because the evidence that it works is overwhelming. However, for those who want to lose weight and stay slim, deciding to try IF as a weight loss mechanism usually requires a deeper understanding. Continue reading to learn why intermittent fasting is so effective and how our bodies react to a longer-than-average fasting window.

2

SCIENCE DOESN'T LIE

Once you have to start counting calories, it takes away from the joy of eating.
–Mireille Guiliano

It is not a coincidence that most Americans have turned toward IF as their weight loss tool. The fact is, it works better than other diets that they've tried. There are several reasons IF works beside it being an incredibly easy lifestyle adjustment to make. Here we'll outline more of what science has told us about what happens on a cellular level when we fast.

WHAT THE MICE SAY

A study conducted in 2012 involved two groups of genetically identical mice in which one group was allowed to eat all day while the second group was restricted to eight hours to consume their meals. Both groups were given the same amount of calories to consume each day. The results showed, after only 18 weeks, that the mice who were allowed to eat all day showed signs of insulin resistance and liver damage. They also weighed 28% more than those on the time-restricted diet.

Then, to address any lingering doubts, the mice that were allowed to eat all day were switched to the time-restricted diet. After the switch, the mice showed improvements in their health and their weight and were able to maintain the weight loss for the duration of the experiment. Scientists also found that these mice had an increased insulin sensitivity.

Some interesting findings from the studies were that even when the mice were given the "weekend off," they still weighed less than the mice who were unrestricted throughout the week. Also, when the eating window was reduced, the mice gained even less weight. The combined findings were unarguably fascinating... but the subjects were unarguably *rodents*.

STUDIES ON HUMANS

In 2015, a study was conducted where a small group of people was asked to restrict their eating windows to a 10-12 hour time frame. They were not given any diet restrictions on what they could eat during that time frame. After 16 weeks, the average weight loss was about eight pounds but the participants reported better sleep, higher energy, and reduced hunger at night. The group also reported that the changes they made to restrict their eating window were easy to implement and sustain.

Satchin Panda is a researcher and professor of circadian biology at the Salk Institute for Biological Studies in La Jolla, California. He has spent most of his career studying the biochemical process of the human body. So far, the subjects of his studies have been mice and people and including the study mentioned above. Other studies that he has conducted have focused on time-restricted eating and produced compelling results. In one study, he asked men at risk of type-2 diabetes to reduce their eating window to ten hours. After twelve weeks, the participants lowered their total cholesterol by 11%. Impressively, after checking in on the participants of the study a year later, 75% of them were voluntarily restricting their eating window to 8-11 hours.

Other researchers have been motivated to find out more since Panda's published studies and have furthered the research on the benefits of IF. One such study was published in *Cell Metabolism* and reported that people who restrict their eating window also reduce their caloric intake unintentionally and end up losing some weight. An analysis of 25 IF studies that were published in the *Annual Review of Nutrition* stated that regardless of the IF method chosen, (there are quite a few and we'll cover the options in another chapter), participants can reduce their overall body weight which aligns with findings from traditional dieting. But in addition to the weight loss, participants consistently showed a decrease in blood pressure, higher insulin sensitivity, and lower cholesterol and triglyceride levels. The most impressive finding was that those who chose to fast using the 5:2 or alternate day fasting methods were able to reduce their body weight by 7% and maintain the weight loss for over a year. For a person weighing 180 lbs, that equates to a loss of 12.5 lbs!

There is unarguably more research needed on all of the benefits of IF on humans; for example, does the human body respond similarly to mice in absorbing less sugar and fats from foods when eating windows are restricted? Does IF protect our brains from degenerative diseases the way it does in mice? Even with these answers not yet discovered for certain, the benefits of IF on humans that have been discovered so far are encouraging.

THINGS TO REMEMBER

- Most dieting Americans find IF the easiest diet to stick with.
- IF allows you to continue enjoying all the foods you love.
- A small adjustment can produce significant changes.
- The benefits of IF go beyond weight loss.

- Studies on humans show that IF can reduce body weight by 7% in a year.

While the benefits in this chapter are for everyone, it is important to note that there are even more benefits of IF specifically for women and men over the age of 50. The next chapter will highlight what makes this method of weight loss the most productive choice for this age group as well as discuss risks they need to be aware of.

3

BENEFITS FOR PEOPLE OVER 50
(AND POSSIBLE RISKS)

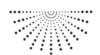

Hitting the 50-year mark is not easy for most of us. I know this well now that I am in my 60's. The days of staying up all night eating junk food and not gaining an ounce (remember your teen years :)) are long gone and our metabolism has become so slow that it feels like its' working backward. This is where IF comes to the rescue with a plethora of benefits geared toward reversing some signs of again all while helping to shed unwanted pounds.

WHAT WE ARE ALL HERE FOR: WEIGHT LOSS

The main driving force behind choosing any diet program is to lose weight. Aspects of a diet plan that increase successful and sustainable weight loss are the ability to stick with it and being able to see and feel the results. Considering IF does not restrict what someone is 'allowed' to eat, it is much easier to commit. In a matter of weeks, people that follow IF eating patterns saw the scale drop by about .5-lbs to 1.5-lbs per week as well as a 4-7% reduction in their waistline. With belly fat being the hardest to lose and a known contributing factor to cardio-vascular disease, it's no wonder why IF is so popular.

The mechanisms that make IF so effective are simple. When we consume our food, enzymes in our gut break down the molecules that eventually end up in our bloodstream. Carbohydrates including sugars and processed grains are deconstructed into sugars and used for energy. If any sugars go unused, they are stored in the fat cells, thanks to insulin. When we allow enough time for the insulin levels in our blood to drop, the sugars are released from the fat cells and burned for energy instead.

One common complaint that people have is that they lose muscle along with fat when they diet. However, a scientific review has shown that reducing eating windows resulted in weight loss with only a 10% reduction in muscle mass versus 25% muscle loss with calorie-restrictive diets.

Likely the most loved benefit of choosing an IF weight loss program is the simplicity of the "rules". Within reason, there are no lists of foods that are off-limits but clean eating is encouraged. And, the concept is easy. Several different eating window time frames can accommodate anyone. Even if someone only restricts the time to eat for the day by a couple of hours, results will be seen.

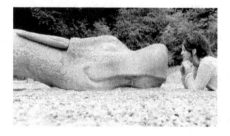

Anti-Aging

Menopause marks an aging milestone that women can't fight no matter how hard they may try to turn back the clock. However, there are ways to prolong some of the changes experienced from aging, through IF. Studies are showing that fasting can slow down the deterioration of cells and their DNA. With cell deterioration being a leading cause of several conditions that become more prevalent as we age, taking steps to keep our cells and DNA healthy can, in theory, offer anti-aging benefits.

Inflammation and cell damage lead to conditions such as heart disease, diabetes, and cancer. When an individual is fasting several cellular changes have been observed. Cells can remove more waste from the tissues. Genes are expressed that prevent disease and prolong the life of the cell. Insulin levels drop and the body's sensitivity to this hormone increases. Inflammation throughout the body is reduced. The body is better able to protect itself against the oxidative stress of free radicals. IF has also been shown to greatly reduce abdominal fat which is a major contributing factor to chronic diseases that shorten one's lifespan.

Another anti-aging benefit of IF is that it supercharges the metabolism. By allowing for larger fasting windows, the body burns more calories more efficiently. This means that when we do eat, essential nutrients in food are more readily accessible to the body. A faster and more efficient metabolism ultimately leads to a healthier and 'happier' body.

Enhanced Mental Health

Fasting has also been shown to enhance the microbiome of the gut (or bacteria in the stomach). Healthy stomach bacteria leads to greater nutrient retention and waste removal. Optimal gut bacteria improves physical and mental health while also contributing to better sleep, memory, and cognition.

As an added benefit, studies have been reported that fasting increases the neuroplasticity of the brain. It has been used to help repair brain damage from strokes or injuries by promoting new neural connections and lowering inflammation. The new neural connections mean that the brain is able to retain new information (learn new things and improve memory). It is also used to lower the risk of developing degenerative diseases of the brain such as Alzheimer's, dementia, and Parkinson's.

In case of women, if menopause has depleted their energy, IF may be the best dieting option for getting that energy back! The energy that is normally used to break down food throughout the day, and into the night, is accessible when fasting. People report having more energy when fasting. This is true both physically and mentally. With cell waste cleaned out, people who fast report feeling rejuvenated and having mental sharpness that they didn't experience previously.

Better Sleep

A common complaint of most of us getting older is that we have a hard time sleeping. Whether it is because of the hot flashes, restlessness, or aches and pains, sleep can be hard to come by as we age. However, research shows that fasting helps to reinforce the body's circadian rhythm. This is important because our circadian rhythm is responsible for various biological functions including our sleep-wake cycle. While the primary contributor to setting the circadian rhythm is sunlight, the secondary contributor is food consumption. Fasting has been shown to increase levels of human growth hormone (HGH) which is produced while we sleep and helps burn fat. In addition to being a magnificent fat-burner, HGH also helps tissues repair themselves and restores muscles. It is responsible for that refreshed feeling we get after a good night's sleep.

Studies are showing that improvements in sleep can occur after only one week of practicing IF. Participants reported that they woke up less at night, and were less fidgety or restless. The studies also showed that participants experienced more rapid eye movement (REM) sleep. REM sleep contributes to our ability to mentally and emotionally process. Participants had improved moods, and overall sleep quality, and were able to focus better during their waking hours.

OTHER BENEFITS

Preventing Dementia

While plenty of clinical trials in mice have shown that IF promotes longevity, a reduction in cognitive deficits, an increase in the production of new brain cells, and improved cognition, human trials are yet to come. Still, observational evidence of human fasting from small, randomized, and controlled studies are suggesting that fasting in humans protects from diabetes and cardiovascular disease which are both associated with a higher risk of dementia. Recent research that looked closely at the connection between dietary patterns and vascular dementia found evidence that fasting could be used as a treatment for preventing the onset of dementia. The theory is that because caloric restriction promotes the suppression of inflammation in the brain, increases insulin sensitivity in the brain, and better controls metabolic energy the effects can protect the brain from the onset of dementia.

Preventing Diabetes

Scientists have confirmed research that IF increases the body's sensitivity to insulin and thus lowers blood sugar. This helps protect against type-2 diabetes and fatty liver. Studies on mice have shown that IF reduces pancreatic fat as well which can also contribute to type-2 diabetes. Other type-2 diabetes preventative outcomes of IF include improved B cell function which helps to lower blood pressure and reduce oxidative stress.

Arthritis

Restricting calories has been shown to have an anti-inflammatory effect on the body. A study published in 2021 revealed relief from Rheumatoid Arthritis (RA) when the participants fasted for 30 days from dawn until dusk for a minimum of twelve hours. The benefits were reported to have lasted up to three months after participants stopped fasting. Also worth mentioning is the reported relief from RA with significant weight loss, lower blood pressure and lower blood sugar... all of which IF addresses. Researchers are also finding a reduction in inflammatory cells, and monocytes, in the blood of people and mice who practice IF. These findings make IF an attractive tile diet option for symptomatic relief of arthritis.

Multiple Sclerosis

A few studies are reporting that IF might provide relief of multiple sclerosis symptoms by inducing a calming effect on the immune response that causes nerve damage. Studies have been conducted in mice where IF contributed to improved gut bacteria and resulted in lower inflammation throughout the body.

Heart Health

According to an endocrinologist at Lenox Hospital in New York, Minisha Sood, a reduction in inflammation in the body contributes to a lower risk of a cardiac event. She states that when the conditions of the microenvironment in the blood vessels favor harmful cholesterol then it results in plaque build-up. The plaque build-up is what causes damage to blood vessels and leads to potentially fatal heart conditions. So, if we can reduce inflammation and change the conditions of the microenvironment within our blood vessels for the better, then we can improve our heart health through IF. One researcher, Dr. Benjamin Horne, compared the effects of fasting to a class of drugs called sodium-glucose cotransporter 2 inhibitors. They lower diabetes and heart failure risk as well as raise the level of a protein in the blood called galectin-3, which reduces inflammation.

Autophagy

Cellular molecule recycling, or autophagy, is a naturally occurring process that assists with cleaning up and renewing cells in the body. It helps to protect against damage such as harmful protein clumps that can lead to neurodegeneration (or loss of neuron function in the brain that can lead to Alzheimer's and Parkinson's disease). While an improvement of this process has been seen in multiple animal studies, one newer human study has also shown promising results. The study's participants had an observed increase in autophagy-related gene expression after only four days of time-restricted eating (IF). This benefit of IF is so important because autophagy increases one's lifespan, protects mental health, deters Alzheimer's, and fights infectious diseases by targeting and destroying foreign bacteria and toxins in our cells.

Cancer

Several researchers have found that fasting has several benefits to protect against and potentially reduce the risk of cancer. Several researchers in San Diego have found that fasting for at least 13 hours per day can help prevent breast cancer from being fatal as well as prevent it from recurring. Several scientists from multiple California universities found that fasting helped reduce the risk of cancer and improved the benefits of cancer treatments. They stated that cells were more receptive to the chemotherapy, protecting normal cells, and promoting cell production. In mice, researchers found that the fasting mice were able to regenerate their immune systems more than non-fasting mice.

POTENTIAL RISKS

As with all diets, there are risks to IF that should be considered before starting. A physician should be consulted so that the right plan, and safest plan, can be mapped out concerning any ongoing conditions. And, if any new conditions arise that are compromising your health, stop fasting and consult a doctor immediately. The following risks are those that were reported as being the most common in IF. They should not be considered as all-inclusive of potential risks with fasting of any kind.

Overeating

For people that have struggled with overeating in the past, binge eating could be a side effect of IF. Going long periods without eating can trigger the urge to eat as much as possible when the eating window begins. This is not the intention of IF and could produce significant problems such as weight gain, feelings of guilt, and possibly even bulimia. It is important to follow a normal eating pattern during the eating windows to avoid overeating or binge eating.

May Affect Certain Medications (Talk to Your Doctor)

It is extremely important to consult your physician about the intention of starting an IF diet if you're currently taking any medications. Whether they are prescribed or over-the-counter, fasting can alter their effectiveness, and absorption rate, and have negative side effects. Some medications need to be taken with food because they are best absorbed with a fat source in the belly or they could produce symptoms of nausea, bloating, and gas on an empty stomach. Other medications are more readily absorbed when fasting. Regardless of the risk or benefit, the prescribing physician should give direction as to whether fasting is safe to do while taking medications.

May Make You Feel Sick

Some people can experience uncomfortable feelings while fasting such as dizziness, nausea, and headaches. When starting an IF diet, the fasting window should only be moderately altered from what the body is already used to. Low blood sugar can feel awful and can be dangerous if fasting is done too aggressively in the beginning. If any of these mentioned symptoms persist with gentle IF or long-term fasting, a physician should be consulted and the diet should be stopped immediately.

MARK'S JOURNEY

"Eventually, I decided that IF was worth trying. I realized that I was already fasting from about 8 p.m. until about 7 a.m. (a full 11 hours regularly). So all I needed to do was stretch that fasting window out a little bit to start seeing some of the benefits that everyone was talking about. I decided to try IF and while the weight didn't drop off immediately, it proved to be a method that was doable and effective. It wasn't long before I even found myself enjoying it. Eventually, I was feeling so good that I knew this wouldn't be a diet for me. It would be a lifestyle."

— MARK, 62 YEARS OLD

THINGS TO REMEMBER

- IF can have an anti-aging effect that specifically addresses the woes of women (and men) over 50.
- The primary benefit of IF has sustained weight loss but there are loads of other benefits too!
- The risks of developing certain diseases increase as we age but IF can contribute to resilience and longevity.
- Sleep gets harder to come by as we age, and is particularly difficult for women in menopause. IF can help with those sleepless nights!
- There are risks involved with IF so be sure to talk to your doctor before you get started.

Knowing the mechanisms behind how IF works helps to decipher what method of fasting is best for each individual. There are a plethora of methods to choose from and depending on your goals, previous experience dieting, and current lifestyle, there will likely be one that outshines the rest for you. Read on to the next chapter to learn more about the different approaches to IF as well as the pros and cons of each.

4
DIFFERENT TYPES OF IF, YOU'VE GOT OPTIONS

Before breaking down the different types of IF, let's first talk a little bit about the first meal that is eaten after a fast… often referred to as 'breakfast.' Most people don't realize that they are fasting everyday and that breakfast was doing exactly what it describes; breaking your fast. Knowing that IF could be just a slightly extended version of what you normally would do is encouraging. This chapter will describe all the different ways to fast and the appropriate ways to break that fast to maximize the benefits.

RESTRICTED EATING WINDOWS

While different methods of fasting are available for a range of lifestyle and dietary needs, all of the fasting options have some general rules of thumb to follow. These 'rules' can be thought of more as exceptions that allow more comfort and ease in maintaining a successful fast.

- First and foremost, calorie-free drinks are allowed during fasting hours because they do not disturb the fasting process. They can help to curb the appetite when in a fasting window.

- IF is most effective with a balanced diet. Making sure to consume all of the proteins and nutrients that the body needs can help with satiating the appetite when it's time to fast.
- When the body fasts, it enters a state of ketosis and burns fat. Fasting is necessary for at least 12 hours to enter ketosis.
- Lastly, sleeping hours count toward fasting hours. This means you can burn fat while resting!

16:8

The 16:8 IF method is the most popular, likely because it is easy to implement immediately into a busy schedule while still having a large impact on healthier living. It encompasses the eating hours to 8 hours. For a lot of people, it provides the perfect balance between getting in a longer fast while still being able to consume food during a large part of their waking hours. For instance, if you finished dinner around 6 pm, you would be able to 'break' your fast at 10 a.m. the next morning. That is plenty of time to drink a cup or two of black coffee or tea to wake you up and get you going for the day.

To start, choose an eating window that works best for you. The time slots can be adjusted, if necessary. And, some people find it helpful to set a reminder on their phone as to when to go into their fasting window and eating window. When you do eat, try filling up on foods that are nutrient-dense with plenty of protein and fiber to keep the appetite at bay during a fast.

Try eating fruits such as berries, citrus, apples, and bananas. Vegetables such as broccoli, cabbage, cauliflower, lettuces, and cucumbers are all great sources of vitamins and fiber. Whole grains such as barley, quinoa, rice, and oats will keep you full by burning slowly. Eat plenty of healthy fats such as olive oil, avocados, and fish. And lastly, protein is a must and can be found in sources such as meat or other options like legumes, nuts, seeds, and eggs.

14:10

The 14:10 method of IF allows for a ten-hour eating window while the other 14 hours of the day are fasting hours. This schedule is great for people who are prone to eating late into the evening. It gives some structure and limitations around a healthier eating schedule while not being too restrictive. It is also a great option for people who started with the 16:8 method but found it to be too difficult. The most popular eating windows for this diet are between 8 a.m. or 9 a.m. and around 6 p.m. or 7 p.m. For most people, this would only stretch their normal fasting hours by a couple of hours which is a great way to start IF.

A study published in *Cell Metabolism* researched a group of people using the 14:10 IF method for about three months. It found that even when people ate whatever they wanted, they unintentionally ate about 8.6% fewer calories, lost 3% of their body weight, and had a loss of 4% of their visceral fat. Visceral fat lines the organs and is a contributor to a variety of major diseases. Blood pressure and cholesterol levels improved as well as their quality of sleep. It was a small change in their lifestyles that led to big health improvements that were easy to sustain.

For anyone needing to start a diet very slowly, maybe due to a doctor's recommendation, the 14:10 diet is a great option. As some time on the 14:10 diet goes by, the next step in shedding a few more pounds might be to include healthier eating options instead of eating pre-diet foods. Also, the 14:10 method can be used as a stepping stone for anyone who feels their weight loss with this method has plateaued. Bumping up the challenge to the 16:8 method might be just what your body is looking for to continue your weight loss journey.

12:12

The 12:12 IF model is much like the previous two mentioned, except the eating and sleeping windows are of equal duration. This is considered the easiest fasting method to start with if your natural eating window is larger than twelve hours in duration. It can be difficult to make lifestyle changes versus what could be viewed as a short-term diet. Living the IF 12:12 method can be a long-term lifestyle change that doesn't require a lot of time, effort, or planning.

A personal trainer and blogger that tried the IF 12:12 method found that it reduced bloating she didn't even know that she had. Even though she is a fitness professional, she acknowledged that not eating first thing in the morning was difficult at first. Starting slowly with the 12:12 method helped her achieve a full 21-day diet plan. And, though she has long since completed her diet program, she still lives a 12:12 IF lifestyle because of all of the health benefits it provides. The biggest change that she reported was that it caused her to think about what she was eating and put a stop to a bad habit of mindlessly snacking. A simple change brought about mindfulness that resulted in big health benefits.

20:4

The 20:4 method of IF is often referred to as the "Warrior Diet" and was first created by Ori Hofmekler in 2001. He calls the 20:4 IF method the Warrior Diet because it is based on the idea that hunters and gatherers only spent a small window of their day eating. Because this IF method is fairly extreme, it is not recommended that anyone should *jump* into it. It's best to start with a more gradual fasting plan and allow the body to adjust before attempting to fast for 20 hours.

It is important to note that this method is different from other IF time-restricted methods that we've mentioned so far because some foods can be consumed during the fasting window. This method also differs from other time-restrictive IF methods because it encourages the participant to schedule their eating window in the evening. A common eating window for the Warrior Diet is from 6 pm until 10 pm. There are also weekly phases to follow if the goal is to work up to this method versus those mentioned so far that can be started immediately.

To begin the weekly phases toward 20:4 fasting, first, start with a detoxing week. During the 4-hour eating window, eat a large salad, several servings of plant proteins, whole grains, cooked veggies, and cheese. During the 20-hour fast, keep calorie intake to a minimum but eating eggs, bone broth, cottage cheese, uncooked fruits, and vegetables, as well as vegetable juices, can help to suppress the appetite and keep blood sugar regulated.

During the second week of the Warrior Diet, the goal is to consume more high-quality fats and fewer carbohydrates. During the 4-hour window, eat meals of lean animal protein, cooked vegetables, nuts, and a large salad with dressing. During the fasting window, eat the same foods mentioned in the detoxing week except add in plain greek yogurt as needed.

The third week of the Warrior Diet consists of alternating high carb and high protein days. For the high carbohydrate days, consume the same foods as in week two during the eating window but add in potatoes, pasta, or oats. On the high protein days, also consume the same foods as in week two except add in 227-454 grams of animal protein as well as some low-carb cooked vegetables.

Once all three weeks of the Warrior Diet have been completed, Hofmekler recommends a second 3-week round of Warrior Diet prep before attempting the 20:4 guidelines. It may be enough, depending on personal weight loss goals, to only follow the 20:4 diet three or four days a week.

Some tips for success that Hofmekler has relayed to those wanting to try any IF diet is listed here:

- Decide when the eating window will be before you start.
- Identify what health goals you're trying to achieve and write them down.
- Put a date on the calendar as to when the diet will start.
- Stick to it for at least 2 weeks.
- Call a friend or health professional for encouragement if it starts to get overwhelming.
- Drink a lot of clear liquids to stay hydrated.

- Eat protein-rich meals later in the eating window.
- Try to eat unprocessed foods.
- Exercise when possible during the fasting window.
- Eat slowly and with the intention of nourishing the body.
- Stay busy to distract from the clock ticking during a fasting window.

Keep in mind that the 20:4 IF method is not for everyone. Some studies have shown weight loss and reduced risk of cardiovascular disease with this diet but it can also come with increased risks. Some things to look for while on the Warrior Diet are brain fog, insomnia, weakness, irritability, stress, anxiety, nutritional deficiencies, and hormonal disruptions. If any of these conditions are presenting themselves, consult a physician because it may be time to either change the duration of your fasting window or stop IF altogether.

5/2

This method of fasting is also known as the "Fast Diet." The general rule of thumb is to eat normally for 5 days and then restrict intake to 500 calories for the other two days of the week. To start the 5:2 diet, choose two fasting days that are non-consecutive during the week. During the fasting days, only eat two or three small meals that are rich in protein and fiber as this will satiate the appetite best throughout the day.

It is important to note that if calorie consumption increases during the non-fasting days then it is unlikely that the diet will be successful. *The goal is to eat normally on the non-fasting days* and cut calories for only two days of the week. Short bursts of willpower are much easier to accomplish than long-term dietary restrictions.

Studies have shown that the 5:2 IF method is an effective weight-loss tool and maintains similar benefits to the other IF methods. Celebrity Jimmy Kimmel gives credit to the 5/2 diet for his 25-pound weight loss. One study reported that participants who fasted in a 4/3 pattern, categorized as *normal* weight and *over*weight, both showed improvements in several areas:

- weight loss of over 11 lbs
- fat loss of over 7.5 lbs (no change in muscle mass)
- Twenty percent lower blood triglycerides
- increased LDL particle size (an improvement)
- reduced inflammation

Eat Stop Eat

This method of IF essentially consists of an eating schedule where a person chooses one or two days (non-consecutive) of the week where they fast for a full 24 hours. The method was developed by Brad Pilon who authored the book *Eat Stop Eat*. While the method is relatively straightforward, the inspiration behind it differs from typical weight loss plans. Pilon emphasizes intentional reevaluation of daily consumption. His thought process involves being mindful and reflecting on what is eaten to make more sensible choices about what we feed our bodies.

The Eat Stop Eat method follows a strict schedule of fasting for a full 24-hour period, but no longer, twice a week. That means that if the fasting day starts at 8 am on Monday, and goes until 8 a.m. on Tuesday, it is important to eat a meal just before the first fasting hour starts and be prepared with a nourishing meal when the 24-hour period ends on Tuesday. Pilon strongly encourages proper hydration on fasting days with clear, calorie-free, fluids.

This method of weight loss focuses on utilizing the body's ketogenic state to burn fat after the first 12 hours of fasting. Unfortunately, everyone reaches this state after different periods and therefore cannot fully rely on reaching ketosis during 24 hours. Also, there can be some greater risks to fasting for a full 24 hours versus IF methods. Some of these risks include symptoms of low blood sugar and some hormonal changes. And, while some hormonal changes can be for the better (possibly increase infertility), others can be very harmful. Other risks are an impulse to binge eat when the 24-hour fasting window expires and some negative psychological impacts including loss of libido and irritability. As always, it is important to consult a physician before starting a new diet, including the Eat Fast Eat method.

Alternate Day Fasting

This method is very similar to the 5/2 IF method except that the fasting days occur every other day. It may be easier for some people to stick with than Eat Fast Eat diet because it allows the consumption of 500 calories on the fasting days. However, it is still fairly restrictive as it requires one or two additional fasting days per week than the 5/2 method.

Studies have researched the effectiveness of the Alternate Day Fasting (ADF) method on adults that were classified as being overweight or obese. Collectively, the participants lost between 3% and 8% of their body fat within 2-12 weeks. The success of this diet was on par with traditional calorie-restrictive diets while allowing one to eat normally every other day.

ADF has been researched by scientists and shown to compare with most calorie-restrictive diets while also having some of the added benefits of other IF methods mentioned. Some findings were from studies ranging from 8-52 weeks where individuals were initially classified as obese or overweight and included the following benefits:

- 2-2.8 inch reduction in waist circumference
- Lower blood pressure
- 20-25% lower LDL (*bad*) cholesterol with an increase in large particle size and a decrease in the more dangerous small LDL particles
- 30% decrease in triglycerides

It is important to realize that ADF is a drastic change from normal eating for most of us and should only be attempted after thorough preparation and full disclosure to a physician. If at any point uncomfortable symptoms arise, stop fasting immediately and talk to your doctor about the best way to proceed with your weight loss goals.

KOOROSH'S JOURNEY

"Initially, I tried the 12:12 method and found that it was a little too easy and did not give me the results I was looking for. I admittedly got a little ahead of myself and decided to try the alternate-day fasting method. While I was able to get through it, I found that I wasn't encouraged to change my entire lifestyle to fit that IF method. Finally, I switched to the 16:8 method and was happy about how quickly I was able to reach my weight loss goal. I was feeling so good on this IF schedule that I dedicated myself to incorporating it into my life permanently."

— KOOROSH, 61 (THE AUTHOR OF THIS BOOK)

THINGS TO REMEMBER

- All IF options outlined include an eating window and a fasting window. Pick the plan that works best for you!
- Don't jump into any IF plan without talking with your physician first.
- Plan a day to start your program and set reminders for your eating and fasting windows.
- Drink plenty of fluids during the fasting windows. Remember that clear fluids are okay to drink during any IF method's fasting windows!
- Set goals for yourself and stick to the IF method that makes the most sense for your goals and your lifestyle.

Now that we've covered the different ways to go about IF, it's time to talk more about how to get started. With beginning a new diet, or eating lifestyle, it is important to set intentions for the greatest chance of success. In the next chapter, we'll discuss all the things to consider so that you can get off on the best foot toward your weight loss journey.

HELP OTHERS FIND THIS BOOK

Science has shown that when you do something nice for someone else, it gives you and the other person a good feeling. This is the easiest way that kindness to strangers pays off. I would like to give you an opportunity to perform an act of kindness during your reading (or listening) experience.

People judge a book by the number of good reviews it has received. The only way for this book to reach many other readers who need it is to have as many reviews as possible.

If you have found this book to be of value so far, would you please take a moment right now and leave an honest review of this book and its contents? It will cost you nothing but it will help one more person who needs this book, find it and use its content to have a healthier and more active life.

This will take you less than a minute of your time. All you have to do is to leave a review.

This will also help this first-time writer.

Please go to the page on Amazon (or where you purchased this book) and leave a review.

Thank you for your kindness.

Now, let's get back to the rest of this book.

5

TIPS FOR GETTING STARTED

The idea of fasting can be intimidating. Nobody *enjoys* feeling hungry. Luckily there are some tips and tricks that will make your IF journey a little easier. With the right frame of mind to equip you for success, IF can be an exciting and transformative process. This chapter will focus on how to prepare for the best IF experience possible.

UTILIZE YOUR SLEEPING HOURS

Going ten or more hours without eating can seem impossible. And it's true that if all fasting hours were also waking hours, IF could seem like torture. However, your sleeping hours count toward fasting as well! We all fast when we sleep so adding on a bit of time in the evening and the morning helps pass the hours of fasting effortlessly.

PLAN AHEAD

Once you've decided on the method of IF that you'll be starting with, it is important to make a plan that you know you can commit to. Map out your fasting window and utilize your sleeping hours as much as possible. Make an effort to meal plan so that you can consume foods that will satiate your appetite throughout the fasting period. By planning how many meals and what they consist of throughout the day you can eliminate mindless snacking and reduce the number of refined sugars and simple carbs that are consumed. It's too easy to hit the drive-through when we're in a hurry and need to grab a quick bite. Instead, have something ready-to-go that is healthy and is just as satisfying as fast food.

Note that if extra calories are eaten during the eating window than would normally be consumed then you can actually gain weight while IF. For example, if you fast for 16 hours and skip breakfast in the morning, don't add an extra meal into the afternoon to "make up for it." The idea is that by fasting, fewer calories will be consumed and weight will ultimately fall away. Be sure not to sabotage your efforts by packing in extra snacks or meals that you would normally eat at that time of the day.

Here is one example of a food, fasting, hydration, and sleep plan that works for long-time intermittent faster Lacey Baier.

6:45 a.m.–9 a.m.: 48-96 oz of water or other calorie-free liquid and gym session

10 a.m.–11:30 a.m.: 1-2 cups of black coffee and more water

11:30 a.m.: Combination of breakfast and lunch with a meal consisting of a toasted muffin with butter, a breakfast burrito, and a portion of berries.

3 p.m.: A big snack consisting of protein pancakes and a protein smoothie.

4 p.m.: A small dinner made up of another wrap. Avocado, turkey, and hummus are one of her favorite, and healthy, combinations.

This plan may seem a bit extreme for anyone that is used to eating dinner later at night or has a habit of snacking after dinner. It isn't designed for everyone! However, it does give an idea of what a successful eating window looks like. Later in this book, we'll cover recipes that you can use to create a meal plan that works best for your personalized IF method.

DON'T STRESS—LISTEN TO YOUR BODY

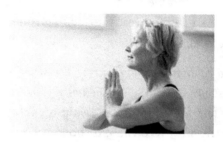

Starting an IF plan that is too aggressive without easing into it can have some counter-productive, and even harmful, effects. It is important to listen to your body for signs that it's time to take a step back and ease into an IF plan a little more gently. Fasting for too long or for too many days per week can alter hormones in the body that will work against your efforts to lose weight. It can slow the metabolism down enough that weight loss slows or even stops during the diet. It can also produce irritability toward those we love. And, for women, it can alter hormones in a way that can be dangerous to your health. During IF there should not be a loss of energy. If there is, then taking a break from IF might be the best option. You can always try again once your system has bounced back with a more gentle approach.

STAY BUSY

Another tip from IF professionals is to keep a busy schedule. Distraction works wonders for passing the time during fasting hours when we're awake. Try getting into a workout routine, get some chores done around the house, or plan an outing with friends or family. Just keep in mind not to put yourself in a situation where it will be more tempting to break your fast earlier than planned.

You may notice that at times of the day when you would typically snack, you're not actually hungry and that you were just doing it out of boredom or habit. IF will help to break those food associations if you work to keep yourself entertained in other ways. Starting an IF plan might be the perfect time to pick up a new hobby or visit the local library for a new book to read. When you're prepping yourself for starting IF, write a list of things that you enjoy doing and start taking steps toward making those more of a priority. That way, not only will your IF journey be more successful, but it will also be enjoyable.

TRACK YOUR PROGRESS

Tracking your progress can help you stick with your IF plan, help build new habits, and showcase the progress you've made. Start with some baseline basics of weight and waist measurements. Then map out a meal plan while also marking the eating and fasting windows of each day. Keep in mind that it can take six to ten weeks to see progress. Average weight loss is about 1-1.5lbs per week but everyone's body is different. If you find that you're losing three pounds per week then you may be cutting too many calories. IF is a dietary change for the long run and is very sustainable once you find a schedule that works for your lifestyle. Tracking your daily progress can help you make adjustments at the beginning that help you stay with the program long-term.

If you're a more tactile-type person, write in a journal to keep notes on how you felt during the day, how well you slept at night, and what meals you consumed at what times of the day. If you're technology-friendly and enjoy the modern-day functionality of apps, take a look at some of these for your IF tracking options:

Window - This app is recommended for "newbie" intermittent fasters. It is user-friendly and tracks all of the important aspects of any IF method. It comes equipped with eating and sleeping window notifications as well as visual graphs so you can see at a glance how well the IF diet is working for you.

Fenometer - Fenometer was specifically designed for women who are using IF as a weight-loss tool. There are options for reminders that can help with hitting weight loss goals, and there are guided tips included with the app.

Fastic - Fastic is a two-in-one app that incorporates the functions of other IF apps but also has added benefits to track meals for better eating as well. There are even recipes that are included!

Zero - This is a customizable IF app that works regardless of the method that you choose. There are template fasting windows included but you also have the option of creating your own. Another perk of this app is that it connects easily with a Fitbit or Oura ring as well.

Fastient - The most unique trait that Fastient boasts above other IF apps are that it allows you to take notes along the way of your fasting journey. There are data entry options that are converted into graphs for an easy to interpret visual of progress. The upgraded version also allows for picture uploads so that you can compare and see the progress for yourself.

BodyFast - This app comes with coaching and meal planning based on various factors entered by the faster. While it does offer more support for IF than most apps, it can also be a bit misleading as it does not contain advice from medical professionals.

Vora - This is a box-standard IF app that incorporates a community of support. Having a group of people that are going through something similar and are willing to partner up can be a bonus for those that need a layer of accountability for their efforts.

DoFasting - DoFasting has a plethora of benefits ranging from over 5,000 recipes to workouts, educational articles, and a platform for creating your meal plan. It also comes with the standard tracking and reminder options that most other IF apps are equipped with.

FastHabit - This app allows you to switch up your fasting schedule at the drop of a hat. If you haven't tried IF before and are not completely sure which method will work best for you, this might be a good app to start with.

LIFE Intermittent Fast Tracker - The LIFE Intermittent Fast Tracker combines many of the same benefits as other IF apps but it also incorporates the addition of eating a Keto diet. The app can tell you when your body may be entering ketosis and it offers a community of support with other people using the app on the same journey.

Ate Food Diary - This app's main feature is that of a visual food diary. Looking back on meals you've made can help associate with what foods make you feel the best. It is also able to post food choices on social media sites.

Simple: Intermittent Fasting - This app boasts having it all! It links up to your iPhone and can track all the usual data as well as your sleeping patterns and water intake. It also contains expert advice and tips to make IF easier.

Fast Tracker: If you're new to fasting, this seems to be one of the easiest fast trackers to use. Simply tell the app when you start and stop eating, and it will track your fasts for you, notifying you when you should start and end fasting according to your schedule.

WHEN TO EXERCISE

Studies are showing that we get the most benefit from a workout that aligns with our natural circadian rhythm. Working out in the morning when we wake up, or as close to it as possible, promotes better sleep quality and maximizes the benefits of improved hormone changes. Digesting food right after a workout can distract the metabolism from prioritizing fat burning during the day. Doing short intervals of high-intensity training can increase testosterone levels, increase brain function, improve body composition, and boost human growth hormone levels. These hormonal shifts can all lead to reduced depression. So ideally, drinking water and working out in the morning a couple of hours before your eating window begins will give you the biggest beneficial outcome while IF.

Even though it is recommended to work out in the morning, it might not be possible for your lifestyle and that's okay! Choose when to work out based on what works best for you. If you can only squeeze in a workout a couple of days a week or only in the evenings, it's still better than not working out at all. Still, it's important to note that the first meal after a workout should be managed with some forethought.

What is the right type of meal to eat after a workout? According to Dr. Nike Sonpal, it is important to eat protein after heavy lifting to support muscle regeneration. And, strength training should be followed with carbohydrates and about 20 grams of protein about a half-hour after working out. However, even the experts won't be able to read what your body needs like you can. Using an app or journal, noting how you feel when you work out in combination with the time frames and meal composition will likely give you the best idea as to what your body feels the best doing and eating.

KATHLEEN'S JOURNEY

> "Before I chose to start IF, I had a fairly set exercise
> schedule that I felt worked well for me. However,
> when I began the 16:8 method, I realized something
> had to change. I wasn't willing to stop IF so my exer-
> cise schedule had to be adjusted. In the past, I had
> found it difficult to exercise first thing in the morn-
> ing. But with IF giving me more energy after a good
> night's sleep, exercising in the morning wasn't as
> difficult anymore. Also, I found that if I got my

workout in earlier in the day, I was able to carry that heightened energy with me until I was ready to go to bed at night. And surprisingly, after a night of fasting, I didn't feel drained in my workouts like I thought I would. The new schedule helped me get through my morning fasting hours and was easier than I thought it would be."

— KATHLEEN, 58 YEARS OLD

THINGS TO REMEMBER

- Utilize your sleeping hours for fasting optimization.
- Plan meals and snacks ahead of time to reduce overeating and mindless snacking.
- Don't stress… listen to your body by tracking your daily eating and sleeping windows as well as your meals and how you felt that day.
- Keep a busy schedule to distract you from a ticking clock during the fasting window.
- Track your progress to stay motivated and engaged in your IF journey.
- Exercise in the morning if you can.

While *what* you eat isn't as crucial to your success with IF as *when* you eat, there are certain foods you can eat to maximize your results. The next chapter will cover why, and how, what you eat matters. We'll discuss certain power foods that can be incorporated into your diet and are delicious! Read on for a look at how what you eat can help you lose weight and be incredibly satisfying.

6

YOU ARE WHAT YOU EAT SO CHOOSE CLEAN EATING

It is true that IF focuses on when you eat versus what you eat as the primary mechanism of losing weight. However as studies have shown, the effectiveness of IF can be increased by eating a cleaner diet. Choosing foods that fuel your metabolism will bring you closer to your weight loss goal faster while helping you feel your best in the process.

Stay Hydrated - While practicing IF, calories that would have been consumed during the fasting hours are cut and so is the water that those foods contained. Considering we get 20-30% of our water from the foods we eat, it is especially important to drink more water while fasting. Proper hydration of the body is what allows cells to function the way they should. Some signs that you may be dehydrated are dry mouth, fatigue, bloating, slow digestion, and thirst. Here are some tips for staying hydrated:

- **First thing in the morning take in 1-2 glasses of water.** This increases your energy levels and speeds up your metabolism. If you frequently wake up at night to urinate or experience heartburn, avoid drinking water shortly before bed.

- **Pay attention to your body's cues.** Pay attention to whether your body is hungry or thirsty. Sometimes we eat too much because we confuse hunger with thirst. Also, examine the color of your urine. Some people monitor their urine's color throughout the day to make sure it is clear or pale. Dark or yellow urine could be a sign of dehydration.
- **Each meal should be preceded by a glass of water.** You'll stay hydrated, have improved digestion of food, and experience fullness more quickly.
- **Take advantage of alarms or notifications.** On your smart devices, set alarms or notifications to serve as reminders throughout the day to drink water. Set your Alexa or Google gadget to remind you and to provide you with verbal, uplifting encouragement as a mental boost.
- **Replace sugary beverages with seltzer or sparkling water.** You'll increase your water consumption in addition to reducing the amount of unneeded sugar you consume.
- **Spend money on a trendy or amusing water bottle.** A decent water bottle can act as a visual prompt to hydrate more frequently throughout the day. Some bottles feature written words of inspiration on the side when the water level drops, or they have marked measurements for tracking consumption.

Coffee - While water is the ideal fluid to drink to stay hydrated, other liquids are also great to drink while fasting. Coffee can help suppress the appetite, increase fat burning, and help reduce insulin. This is what makes coffee a perfect liquid to drink while fasting. Be careful though! Coffee drinks filled with sugar and milk or cream will result in a hard stop of a fast and will stack up the calories quickly. A 20-oz vanilla latte has 510 calories in it! Black coffee contains less than five calories and will not break your fast. Avoid adding extra stuff like milk and sugar because their calorie content will disrupt your ketosis. Some people will have a cup of bulletproof coffee in the morning so they can last until lunch time. However, bulletproof coffee usually contains calorie-enriched ingredients, such as unsalted grass-fed butter or ghee, coconut oil, and sometimes sweeteners and it is considered as a substitute for breakfast because its packed full of calories (around 250 to 500 calories per cup). In other words, you will be breaking your fast by having bulletproof coffee. Stick with black coffee if you don't want to break your fast. Other liquids that can be consumed during a fast are herbal teas, Apple cider vinegar, and pure fats.

Herbal teas have antioxidant properties that can boost fasting processes in the body. It is common to drink green or black tea but that is not all. Here are some other types of tea that you may consider.

- Immortalitea Diet Tea: Fasting Tea For Weight Loss - This fasting tea combines 11 herbs to boost your metabolism and help control hunger. It's a healthy and refreshing mixture of ginseng, ginger, Chinese yam root, red dates, poria, rehmannia, licorice, atractylodes, peony, dogwood fruit, and alisma. You can really taste the variety of flavors in one cup of this tea.
- Yogi Tea: Green Tea Blueberry Slim Life - Yogi "Green Tea Blueberry Slim Life" tea is a mix of green tea, bright hibiscus, and sweet blueberry. It tastes very natural but flavorful at the same time. A great choice for someone looking for a bit of energy boost as it has caffeine from green tea. Additionally, the mix of other ingredients like blueberries and hibiscus gives it a wholesome taste.
- Gaia Herbs: Cleanse & Detox Herbal Tea - Gaia Herbs tea is great if you're looking for detox and weight loss. It's a versatile mix of herbs like rooibos, fennel, aloe vera and others. A nice addition is the lemon and peppermint essential oils. To top it all, the ingredients are organic and caffeine-free. Therefore, this tea can be enjoyed in the evening without worrying about disturbing your sleep.

Preparation of tea: When using loose-leaf tea, it can be difficult to recognize the ratio of tea-to-water that you should be using. To make it simple, you want to use 1-2 teaspoons of premium loose-leaf tea for every 6-8 ounces of water. That means that if your teapot or kettle holds 24 ounces of water, you want to use somewhere around 5 teaspoons of loose-leaf tea.

Brew Method: Once you've measured out the amount of tea you're going to brew, you need to decide how you're going to brew it! A simple method intended for one-time use is to utilize *tea filters*. Just scoop your tea into the filter, place it in your mug or to-go cup, and add hot water. Another easy (and fun) way to brew your herbal tea is to use a *tea infuser*! A tea infuser is a reusable tea filter, making it environmentally friendly and ideal for home usage. Tea infusers come in all shapes and sizes, ranging from super simple metal designs to mana-teas! All you have to do is scoop your desired amount of premium loose-leaf into the infuser, place it in your mug or travel cup, and add hot water. If you're making a batch of tea larger than a single-serving, you can still use tea bags and tea infusers to brew your loose-leaf tea. However, another great idea is to use a French press! If you already have one at home, it eliminates the need for tea filters and infusers and allows you to make a large batch of delicious herbal tea.

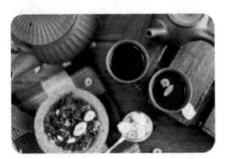

The next step in brewing your perfect cut of herbal tea is determining the amount of time for which it needs to be steeped. This step is critical in creating a great tasting tea. Why? Because steeping your tea for too long can create bitterness, whereas not steeping long enough will leave your tea wanting for more flavor. For an ideal flavor, herbal tea should be steeped for 4-6 minutes at a temperature of 100 degrees Celsius (or 212 degrees Fahrenheit). After about 5 minutes, your tea will be finished steeping and you can remove your tea filter or infuser, then enjoy your cup of tea!

Apple cider vinegar (ACV) helps to lower blood sugar, lowers cholesterol, and can improve weight loss while practicing IF, and can assist diabetics in controlling their blood sugar levels. According to some research, drinking vinegar after a meal high in carbohydrates can increase insulin sensitivity by up to 34% and considerably lower blood sugar. A typical dose is 1–2 tablespoons (15–30 ml) mixed with one cup of water and taken before or after meals.

In addition to taking ACV with water, you can also create a salad dressing with it. Simply add one or two tablespoons to your salad or combine with lemon, olive oil, or any other of your preferred ingredients.

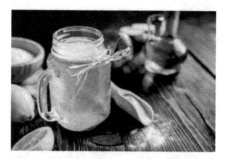

There are situations when using apple cider vinegar to lose weight is advised. This is so that it might make you feel satisfied. If losing weight and reducing belly fat are your goals, several short-term studies have suggested that drinking apple cider vinegar may help you eat fewer calories. However, unless a person also undertakes other dietary and lifestyle adjustments, its long-term benefits for weight loss are uncertain and probably will not be significant.

A couple of other liquids that are perfectly acceptable during a fast are sparkling water, lemon water, and clear broth. The most important thing to remember is to keep liquids as calorie-free and sugar-free as possible.

AVOCADO

Everyone knows that avocados are a superfood but they are especially powerful when paired with IF. They are packed with fiber which helps to keep you feeling full longer and aids in removing waste from the body. They are also packed with almost 20 vitamins and minerals and contain loads of monounsaturated fat (the good kind!). The oils from avocados help reduce pain from arthritis and osteoporosis by lowering inflammation in the body.

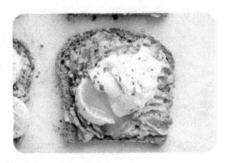

Here is a simple recipe for *Toast with avocado and an egg inside:* Cut out a 2-inch hole from one piece of lightly toasted bread. In a small oven-proof nonstick skillet, heat 1 tablespoon of the oil over medium heat. Add the bread and crack 1 egg into the hole. 2 minutes should be enough time to cook the egg until the bottom begins to set. When the egg white is set but the yolk is still runny, transfer it to the oven and bake for 4 to 5 minutes at 375 degrees F. Around the egg on the toast, spread 1/2 an avocado that has been mashed and seasoned with spicy sauce, salt, and pepper. Add chopped cilantro and chives on top.

Avocados provide a plethora of other benefits such as protecting the eyes from UV light damage, lower inflammation in the heart, reducing blood pressure, and even reducing depression thanks to their high levels of folate. Just keep in mind that avocados are high in calories so a serving should be kept to about a half of one medium avocado. The unique make-up of this superfood can help to suppress hunger and avoid sugar spikes in the blood without having to consume carbohydrates or limit calorie intake.

FISH AND SEAFOOD

Researchers, physicians, and scientists agree that fish is a nutrient-dense superfood that we should all be incorporating into our diets for several reasons. It is filled with omega-3 fatty acids and has loads of other nutrients such as magnesium, potassium, iron, zinc, calcium, and phosphorus. Besides all of these wonderful vitamins and minerals, fish is also high in protein. This makes fish a perfect choice of animal protein during an eating window while practicing an IF method of weight loss.

Besides aiding in weight loss and dietary essentials, fish contributes to a healthier body and lifestyle as well. It can lower the risk of heart attack and stroke. It boosts the functionality of the brain and can help prevent and treat depression. It provides supplementation of vitamin D for people that can't get enough from the sun. Eating fish regularly can reduce the risk of autoimmune diseases such as type 1 diabetes. It has a protective effect on our vision during later years of life. And, eating plenty of fish can improve our quality of sleep.

CRUCIFEROUS VEGETABLES

Cruciferous vegetables are a group of green veggies composed of broccoli, cabbage, kale, bok choy, arugula, Brussel sprouts, collards, watercress, arugula, radishes, and cauliflower. They are all members of the mustard family and have very similar compositions of nutrients and beneficial contributions to the body. They carry a rich store of vitamins A and C as well as minerals such as folate and vitamin K. They also contain phytonutrients which may help to reduce inflammation. They are fiber-dense so aid in feeling satiated without overeating.

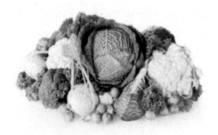

A variety of studies have shown that diets rich in cruciferous vegetables can lower the risk of certain cancers including breast, bladder, lung, prostate, pancreatic, and colon cancer. It seems that there are enzymes within these veggies that protect the DNA from damage. They also have some antioxidant properties that counteract cancer-causing nitrosamines and polycyclic aromatic hydrocarbons (usually a result of charred or cured meats).

POTATOES (THEY GET A BAD RAP!)

Potatoes are surprisingly healthy when they are prepared the 'right' way. Most of us think of potatoes as being bad for us because they contain carbohydrates and are often prepared by fast-food restaurants by being boiled in a vat of oil. In that case, it is understandable that we tend to avoid them. However, potatoes are packed with fiber (specifically, resistant fiber) that causes less gas and bloating than other vegetables. The fiber contained in potatoes acts as a prebiotic for optimal gut health and food digestion. This reduces constipation and irritable bowel syndrome. Potatoes are also high in antioxidants and fight free radicals that can damage cells and lead to cancer. Besides fiber and prebiotics, potatoes also contain vitamin C, and B6, potassium, manganese, magnesium, phosphorus, niacin, and folate.

One study showed that potatoes were ranked as being the most filling common food among 38 different foods. Their ability to fill us up is due to the high fiber content as well as a protein called potato proteinase inhibitor 2 which helps to release hormones that make us feel full. Another benefit of potatoes is that they are naturally gluten-free. They reduce inflammation in the colon and improve our digestive health. And, potatoes can reduce the body's resistance to insulin and thus improve the control of blood sugar levels.

BEANS, BEANS, THE MAGICAL FRUIT

Beans are an excellent source of protein and fiber. They contain amino acids which provide for protein composition. They contain both soluble and insoluble fiber which aids in several bodily systems. They both help to control the appetite by inducing a feeling of fullness. Soluble fiber lowers cholesterol by turning into a gel in the stomach that absorbs LDL (bad) cholesterol. This results in a lower risk of heart disease and stroke. The insoluble fiber helps to feed good bacteria in the gut which helps to keep the digestive system running smoothly, helps to support the immune system, maximizes nutrient absorption, and promotes weight loss.

Beans are rich in folate and they contain loads of antioxidants and anti-inflammatory agents which reduce the risk of cancer. They help to lower cholesterol and the risk of coronary heart disease. Adding beans to the diet can also contribute to the stabilization of blood glucose and help to prevent diabetes and fatty liver.

EGGS

Eggs are a nutrient powerhouse comprised of protein, folate, iodine, carotenes, choline, betaine, and vitamins A, B12, and D. The protein content of eggs consists of all nine essential amino acids which are needed for complete protein. Eggs contain a large portion of protein without carrying a ton of calories which makes them a great diet food. They support weight management effectively because protein is more filling than both fat and carbohydrates. Betaine and choline help support heart health and reduce the risk of stroke and heart disease. Choline is especially precious because it is needed for the cell membranes in brain tissue to allow for proper cell function and normal brain development. Vitamin A is key to maintaining optimal eyesight. Carotenes protect our eyes against macular degeneration and cataracts.

There was a misconception for some time that eggs were not good for you because they are high in cholesterol. However, we know now that they are comprised of large LDL cholesterol particles versus the dangerous small LDL particles. Overall, increasing the particle size of LDL cholesterol in the blood reduces the risk of heart attack and stroke.

For an added benefit, you can now buy eggs that are enriched with omega-3 fatty acids as well. The chickens are fed a specialized diet that fortifies the eggs they lay. The result is that the eggs are rich in omega 3's and, when consumed, aid in reducing the blood triglyceride levels by 16-18%

WHOLE GRAINS

It can be confusing as to what constitutes a "whole grain." However difficult marketing experts try to make it, the answer is simple. Every edible part of the grain must be present, deconstructed, or intact, for something to be considered a whole grain. Examples include whole-grain corn, oats, popcorn, brown rice, whole rye, whole-grain barley, wild rice, buckwheat, triticale, bulgur (cracked wheat), millet, quinoa, sorghum, and 100% whole wheat flour. Nutrients that can be found in whole grains include trace minerals (iron, zinc, magnesium, and copper), protein, fiber, manganese, magnesium, B vitamins, antioxidants, and plant compounds such as polyphenols, stanols, and sterols (these aid in preventing disease).

The benefits of eating whole grains include supporting healthy gut bacteria, optimizing digestion, and encouraging regular bowel movements. Eating whole grains has been shown to lower the chance of developing type-2 diabetes, obesity, heart disease, and some types of cancer. Several studies have shown that the higher the whole grain make-up of total carbohydrates in one's diet, the lower the individual's risk of a heart attack. In a study conducted for 10 years with 1,424 adults, the participants with the highest whole grain intake had as much as 47% lower risk of heart disease. In another study, those who had higher whole grain intake also had a 14% lower risk of stroke.

Beyond the benefits mentioned thus far, studies on whole grain consumption have shown to reduce the risk of colorectal cancer (one of the most prevalent types of cancer). The anti-cancer components of whole grains that we know of so far are fiber and prebiotics. Other components include phenolic acids, phytic acids, and saponins which may slow down the development of cancers.

BERRIES

Berries pack a super-nutrient punch as well with their antioxidant properties and other health benefits. Blueberries, blackberries, and raspberries have the highest level of antioxidants than any other fruits, besides pomegranates. Unstable free radicals are harmful to cells and their damage can lead to cancer. Antioxidants stabilize free radicals thus protecting our cells against said damage and cancer as well as some diseases. Just one cup of blueberries a day has shown to have these protective benefits.

Other health benefits of consuming berries include reduced insulin levels and improved insulin sensitivity, protecting the body against inflammation that contributes to diabetes, heart disease, obesity, and improving the function of arteries and blood vessels. They also lower bad cholesterol levels and improve skin protective collagen levels. One study even showed that those who ate berries regularly could prevent the mental decline that comes with age. The subjects participating in the study had better thinking, reasoning, and memory.

Berries are also high in fiber which aids in satisfying hunger, slows down the digestive tract, and reduces the number of calories consumed from food (up to 130 calories!) throughout the day. In addition to high fiber content, berries are also high in vitamin C (especially strawberries) and consist of many other vitamins and minerals including manganese, vitamin K1, copper, and folate. All of these benefits are included in a single serving, about 3.5 ounces, and only contain about 45 calories!

All of these benefits are truly incredible but the best part about berries is that they taste delicious! They are sweet enough to satisfy a serious sweet tooth but don't affect blood sugar the way other sweets can. They can be added to salads, smoothies, yogurt, and a variety of other dishes, or just eaten all on their own without any preparation. Even out of season, frozen berries work just as well and can be thawed as needed.

NUTS

Nuts have several amazing health benefits including the ability to help us lose weight. A large study found that people who ate nuts resulted in an average of 2 inches lost from the waistline versus other participants who were assigned to eat olive oil instead. Another study showed that people who ate almonds lost three times as much weight as those that didn't. Research shows that though nuts are high in calories, not all of the calories are absorbed in the body thus aiding in a sense of fullness without the full caloric impact. They also aid in lowering bad cholesterol, raising good cholesterol, reducing triglycerides, as well as contributing to maintaining low blood sugar levels resulting in protection against type-2 diabetes and metabolic syndrome. They reduce inflammation as well and promote healthy aging. Brazil nuts, walnuts, and almonds have especially protective properties and are therapeutic for those with serious conditions such as diabetes and kidney disease. These contributions that nuts make to our bodies have shown to be exceptionally beneficial to heart tissue. They reduce the risk of heart attack and stroke.

Besides being delicious and easy to pack around for a quick snack, nuts contain tons of nutrients and health benefits too. They contain protein, monounsaturated fat (the *good* kind), fiber, vitamin E, magnesium, phosphorus, manganese, and selenium. They also have tons of antioxidants. Nuts containing the wonderful benefits mentioned are almonds, pistachios, walnuts, cashews, pecans, macadamia nuts, Brazil nuts, hazelnuts, and peanuts (though these are technically a legume with 'nut-like' properties).

GEORGE'S JOURNEY

"One thing that I was never very disciplined about was my water intake. I knew it was a problem, so with IF I make more of an effort to drink plenty of H2O. So I incorporated a few techniques to help me remember to get the proper intake every day. First, I downloaded an IF app to track and set reminders to drink water throughout the day. I also bought myself a new water bottle that is easy to take with me everywhere I go. Every time it's empty, I make a point to fill it up. Collectively, it has made a huge difference in the amount of water I drink daily and in the success I've had with IF."

— GEORGE, 72 YEARS OLD

THINGS TO REMEMBER

- Eating superfoods while IF can boost weight loss.
- Prepping healthy food for consumption during the eating window can help you feel great throughout the day.
- There are added health benefits to including these foods into your diet besides just weight loss.
- While IF focuses mainly on when you eat versus what you eat, it is never a bad idea to improve your diet as well.
- Many of the superfoods mentioned are readily accessible, inexpensive, easy to prepare (or require no preparation), and incredibly satisfying.

Just think about it this way - Eating well while IF will give you far better results than eating processed foods while trying to lose weight. If you're worried about feeling too hungry during a fast, nutrient-dense food will help you get through it. And adding these superfoods to your diet will have you feeling better than you've ever felt before.

7

MISTAKES AND HOW TO AVOID THEM

I n this chapter, we'll discuss some of the most common mistakes that people make while on their IF journey. Having an awareness of possible pitfalls can help you be mindful of your intentions of sticking with IF. Keep in mind that changing long-term habits can be difficult. But with guidance and dedication, your weight loss goals *are* attainable.

STAY FOCUSED

Focus requires conscious effort but several tools can help. For anyone, it can be exceptionally difficult to stay focused if they're not getting enough sleep. Set yourself up for restful nights as well as you can. Having some warm chamomile tea or a bath in the evening can help you wind down. Think about how successful the day was in your IF journey and be proud of yourself.

During the day, stay busy with work, friends and family, or a new hobby. If activities in the day are planned ahead of time, there won't be as much of an opportunity for lackadaisical snacking or breaking your fast too soon. When in the eating window, ask yourself if you're truly feeling hungry before you eat something. Could you possibly be feeling some emotions that could be soothed in alternative ways from eating? Keeping a journal or meditation may aid the mind's restlessness and provide heightened awareness of what your body is asking you for. Another trick to try is drinking a glass of water before you eat to find out if maybe what you thought was hunger might be thirst or boredom.

Lastly, stay focused by avoiding distractions that can lead you off-track from your IF goals. Celebrating a friend's birthday at a restaurant is an example of a situation that could derail your IF progress or give you a reason to be proud of your dedication to your weight loss goals. Before you go, note how the outing will fall in conjunction with your eating and fasting windows. You can adjust these time frames to allow you to have a meal a bit later than you normally would. Also, try to take a look at the menu online beforehand if possible. There are likely some options that will suit your meal plan but don't be shy to request healthy adjustments when it comes time to order. If an IF distraction comes in the form of a spontaneous trip through the drive-through window, ask yourself if it will be worth the setback.

BE DISCIPLINED

Set measurable goals to help identify the purpose of your IF path. Write down *why* you started IF and reference it frequently. This should not be a list of tasks to complete, but rather deeper reasoning within yourself to motivate you through the journey. Small, attainable, steps can be identified so that it's easier to see when progress is being made. When you complete a step toward your goal, reward yourself and share your success with others.

Be gentle with yourself and know that some days will be harder than others. Know that the hard work you're putting into IF is for yourself. You earn the rewards of IF and you are worthy of them. Share how you're feeling with a community of people who will support you and help you stay accountable for your goals and efforts. If you don't have acquaintances who are using IF, you can go online and find IF groups. There are many IF groups on Facebook, for example. Members of these groups can be very supportive of each other. Sometimes we all need to seek a bit of motivation from outside of ourselves.

Reading articles or blogs of people that have succeeded in similar IF journeys can help you to visualize your healthy future. Note the days that you felt really good and what made them successful, then reference those on days that could've gone better. Above all, stay positive. There is no easy way to change a lifestyle but know that every small change counts. Feels of better balance, confidence, and energy are all wonderful accomplishments that should be acknowledged and celebrated.

EAT THE RIGHT FOODS

If the scale is not moving in the direction you were hoping for, or it just isn't moving at all, it could be because of what you're consuming during the eating windows. *Ultimately, utilizing any IF method should cut calories out of your diet.* However, if you're making up for the breakfast you missed earlier in the day then it could work against you. Be careful not to use IF as a free pass to eat whatever, and however much, you want during the eating window. You could end up watching the scale move in the wrong direction.

If you find yourself 'starving' during the fasting window and then tend to overeat (or binge eat) during the eating window then it's likely you're eating the wrong foods. Eating simple carbohydrates, processed food, and sugar will spike your blood sugar and then send it crashing right back down again. This will set you up for feeling hungry again sooner. Be sure to include lots of fiber, protein, and nutrients in your diet to sustain your appetite for as long as possible.

EASE INTO IT

When starting on IF, don't pick the hardest fasting duration to stick to. Regardless of how much weight you'd like to use, it's best to start slow and allow your body to adjust to the new eating schedule. The first few days are bound to be difficult but shouldn't feel impossible. If you're ready to give up, maybe just take a step back. Widen the eating window by a few hours and don't guilt yourself over the adjustment. Sticking with a slightly more gentle IF plan will still lead to weight loss and will likely have you feeling great in no time.

Be sure to utilize your sleeping hours as best you can as well. If you know that not eating in the evenings is especially difficult for you, shift your eating window so that your fasting awake hours are mostly in the morning. And when you do eat, use a meal plan to incorporate nutrient-dense foods that will see you through the next fast.

CHOOSE THE RIGHT PLAN

So far, studies have shown that there is no general "best plan" for IF. The best plan is the plan that you can commit to and stick with. It is also important to note that there is no bad time to change the plan once you realize that it isn't working in your favor. If you've been successfully doing the 12:12 IF method and are now seeing a stall in your progress, it may be time to move to the 14:10 method. Know what your tendencies are and choose a plan that will cater toward avoiding your weaknesses. If you could never manage to skip breakfast in the morning then don't attempt to follow an IF method where you're faced with holding out until lunch for your first meal of the day. And, don't forget to consult your physician. They will likely have some wise insight on what might be the best plan to start with.

SUSAN'S JOURNEY

"I made a few mistakes when I first started mine IF journey. One mistake that I've found is very common for others starting on IF is that I ate too many calories during my eating window. I was so hungry by the end of my fasting window that I overate as soon as it ended. Then I would load up on calories before the next fasting window began. I was doing it because I didn't think I could refrain from eating for the full fasting window if I didn't make up for those missed calories elsewhere. As it turns out, that logic defeated the purpose of fasting altogether. Instead, I had to shift my food choices to those that would sustain me through the fasting window without feeling like I was starving. After a little practice, patience, and a few adjustments, I can honestly say that I feel better than I ever have."

— SUSAN, 63 YEARS OLD

THINGS TO REMEMBER

- Stay focused on the IF plan that you've chosen.
- Utilize your sleeping hours for your fasting window.
- Stay disciplined by setting goals and determining why you are using IF as a weight nutrient-denseness tool.
- Choose nutrient dense foods that will sustain you through your fast.
- Start slowly and set attainable goals.
- Choose the right plan, schedule the IF days/windows, then ease into it.

IF is unlike any other diet plan because it can be sustained as a lifestyle that leaves you feeling fit and refreshed each day. However, especially in the beginning, it should be started slowly like any other weight loss diet. Starting IF too aggressively can feel defeating and can be dangerous. Work up to the fasting duration that works best for your body and your lifestyle.

8

HOW TO BREAK YOUR FAST

After a successful fasting window, especially a longer one, you may feel like you could eat just about anything in sight. Take a deep breath and remember that you don't want to undo any of your hard work. This chapter will cover the best ways to break your fast so that you don't end up feeling hungry again sooner than necessary.

LOW-CARB, HIGH-FAT

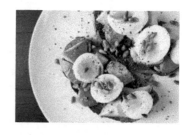

When coming out of a fast, the best way to keep the metabolism operating at optimal levels is to eat a low-carb, high-fat meal. Diet Doctor suggests starting with a large glass of water and then composing a salad of spinach, tomato, and parsley topped with olive oil. Add a protein like chicken or fish the size and thickness of the palm of your hand. Then fill the rest of your plate with above-ground vegetables that are raw or cooked in a natural fat like ghee, butter, coconut, or avocado oil. If you feel like you could still eat a bit more, snack on an avocado.

FRUITS

During a long fast, the lining of the stomach can diminish which can make it difficult to digest certain foods. Thus, breaking your fast with simple and easy-to-digest food like fruit or fruit juices can be a little easier for the stomach to break down. Watermelon, grapes, and apples are easily digested. Start with small bites or sips of juice if it's been a particularly long fast to give the body time to adjust to accepting food again. It's advised to stay away from acidic or spicy foods at first if your tummy tends to be sensitive coming out of a fast.

BONE BROTH

The body tends to lose electrolytes when fasting even if you've been drinking plenty of water. Breaking a fast with bone broth is a great way to restore essential electrolytes such as magnesium, potassium, calcium, and sodium. Organic bone broth can help the gut absorb other nutrients consumed throughout the eating window. Other benefits of breaking a fast with bone broth are that it is easily digestible and won't cause any discomfort to the stomach. It supplies collagen to the skin, muscles, and bones. It has anti-inflammatory amino acids that help improve sleep. It can help calm the gastro-intestinal tract and it will deliver healthy fats without added carbs. And the best part is that it tastes delicious!

APPLE CIDER VINEGAR

There are loads of dietary and health perks that come along with consuming apple cider vinegar (ACV). And, though it does not break your fast, it is beneficial to start your eating window with one or two tablespoons of ACV mixed with a cup of water. Studies have shown that ACV can suppress the appetite and promote feelings of fullness, contribute to weight loss, and improve blood sugar levels. It is recommended that ACV be diluted before consumption because of its high acidity and ability to readily erode tooth enamel. There are pill and gummy forms of ACV that can be a bit easier to take for some people. Also, be sure that ACV is not consumed after the expiration date or it can have several adverse effects.

PROTEIN

Protein is an essential nutrient whether fasting or not. However, it is a particularly helpful nutrient that if consumed when breaking a fast can help ward off hunger and overeating during an eating window while practicing IF. A common "break-fast" could include eggs, cheese, yogurt, smoothies, etc. However, there are some other, less traditional but just as satisfying, means of breaking a fast with a protein-rich meal. Smoked salmon, dinner leftovers, bean burritos, and nut butter on whole-grain toast are all wonderful breakfast alternatives. It is recommended to eat between 15-30 grams of protein in the first meal after a fast to get the best start to consuming enough protein during the eating window.

KOOROSH'S JOURNEY

"Now that I've been practicing a method of IF that works for me, I've begun to focus more on the fuel (food) that I put into my body. The first meal after a fasting window tends to make or break how successful my IF day goes and largely determines how well I feel and how well I sleep. A lot is riding on the first meal of the day for me. So, I try to have a couple of easy staple 'break-fast' foods in the house regularly. Eggs (or eggbeaters) with sautéed vegetables and ground turkey on top of a slice of Ezekiel bread is my usual go to meal straight out of a fast, but you can also switch things up with greek yogurt and fruit at times as well. When I need something more out of the box, I look up new, yummy, IF recipes to whip up."

— KOOROSH, 61 (AUTHOR)

THINGS TO REMEMBER

- There are several ways to break a fast without undoing the hard work put into the fasting window.
- Choosing the right meal to break your fast sets you up for a successful eating window and next fasting window.
- Tend to the stomach with gentle foods and tend to the body with essential nutrients.
- Start with foods that are low in carbs, high in fats, fruits, bone broth, and/or rich in protein.
- ACV won't break your fast but will boost the effects of your IF efforts.

With all the ins and outs of IF now at your fingertips, read on to the next chapter to find recipes that can be used in your meal plan. Chapter 9 outlines breakfast recipes that are IF-friendly, easy to prepare, and guaranteed tasty!

9
CONCLUSIONS

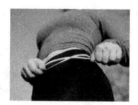

I ntermittent fasting includes many health benefits, including weight loss, enhanced brain function, cancer prevention, and more. With IF, you will find success and a happier, healthier you. Don't let menopause or any other hormonal changes control your weight. IF is your tool to take control of your metabolism and longevity.

It is never too late to start on a path to a healthier lifestyle. In our later years of life, aches and pains become a regular occurrence and something we learn to live with. However, it doesn't have to be that way. We can feel young and vibrant again by simply adding a few parameters to our lives and connecting with a community of support and resources. When we find success and feel our best, we inspire others to do the same. Your journey could spark the start of another's. The ripple effect is a wonderfully strong force that can save our friends, family, and neighbors from unnecessary pain or sadness in their own lives.

For your convenience, I have provided some recipes and a 21-day meal plan in Part II of this book. Start IF *today* and leave a review of this guide so that others can find and utilize these helpful tips, tricks, and recipes!

ACKNOWLEDGMENTS

This book is the fruit of many hours of rewriting and editing. I am proud of the final product and hope that you have enjoyed reading it as well. I would like to thank my wife, Linda for all her help with editing this book, rewriting recipes, and listening to me mull over the different ways this material could be presented and giving me feedback.

I would also like to thank our friend and neighbor, Patti Criswell, for her excellent editorial comments on my first draft. Your comments were on the mark and critical to the success of this book.

My daughter, Mimi, and my step-daughter, Elyse tried out some of the recipes in this book and provided feedback. These comments were excellent and helped improve this book. Thank you!

GLOSSARY

ADF: Alternate day fasting.

Alternate day fasting: The practice of fasting on certain days and eating normally on the others.

Autophagy: Literally 'self-eating'; regulated mechanism of the cell that removes unnecessary or dysfunctional components.

Eating window: The period of time you eat.

Extended fasting: Fasting for longer than 24 hours.

Fasting window: The period of time you don't eat.

Intermittent fasting: The practice of splitting each 24 hour period into an eating window and a fasting window.

IF: Abbreviation for intermittent fasting.

Window: A period of time.

REFERENCES

Appenbrink, Kr. (2020, December 29). *20 Veggie Snacks for Feel-Good Munching.* Kitchn. https://www.thekitchn.com/healthy-vegetable-snacks-233565

Aubrey, A. (2019, December 8). *Eat For 10 Hours. Fast For 14. This Daily Habit Prompts Weight Loss, Study Finds.* NPR.org. https://www.n-pr.org/sections/thesalt/2019/12/08/785142534/eat-for-10-hours-fast-for-14-this-daily-habit-prompts-weight-loss-study-finds#:~:text=For%2010%20Hours.-

Aug. 12, T. P. |. (2020, August 12). *31 Vegetable Snacks That Will Hold You Over Until Dinnertime.* PureWow. https://www.purewow.com/food/vegetable-snacks

Aura, S. (2022, February 3). *20 Fresh and Healthy Fruit Breakfast Recipes.* Tea Breakfast. https://teabreakfast.com/fruit-breakfast-recipes/

Axe, J. (2019, May 1). *How Intermittent Fasting and a Healthy Diet Boost Mental Health.* 24Life. https://www.24life.com/how-intermittent-fasting-and-a-healthy-diet-boost-mental-health/

Baier, L. (2021, October 21). *Intermittent Fasting Meal Plan | How To Create Your Eating Routine*. A Sweet Pea Chef. https://www.asweet-peachef.com/intermittent-fasting-meal-plan/

Ball, D. J. (2021, February 2). *35 Veggie-Packed Dinners in 30 Minutes or Less*. EatingWell. https://www.eatingwell.com/gallery/7822990/veg-gie-packed-dinners-30-minutes/

Berg, E. (2017, December 30). *Getting Enough Nutrients & Calories on Intermittent Fasting ? – Dr.Berg*. Www.youtube.com. https://www.y-outube.com/watch?v=h1hBRLi5QWY

Berger, M. (2019, August 22). *How Intermittent Fasting Can Help Lower Inflammation*. Healthline; Healthline Media. https://www.healthline.-com/health-news/fasting-can-help-ease-inflammation-in-the-body

Bioge. (2020, October 29). *How Intermittent Fasting Can Help to Fight Aging*. BioAge Health. https://www.bioagehealth.com/how-intermit-tent-fasting-can-help-to-fight-aging/#:~:text=Calorie%20restric-tion%20and%20intermittent%20fasting

Bjarnadottir, A. (2018). *The beginner's guide to the 5:2 diet*. Healthline. https://www.healthline.com/nutrition/the-5-2-diet-guide

Bjarnadottir, A., & Kubala, J. (2020, August 4). *Alternate-Day Fasting*. Healthline. https://www.healthline.com/nutrition/alternate-day-fast-ing-guide#basics

Booth, S. (2020, July 14). *Everything You Need to Know About Avocados*. WebMD. https://www.webmd.com/food-recipes/all-about-avoca-dos#:~:text=Avocados%20are%20low%20in%20sugar

Botterman, L. (2021, October 11). *Research review shows intermittent fasting works for weight loss, health changes | UIC Today*. Today.uic.edu. https://today.uic.edu/research-review-shows-intermittent-fasting-works-for-weight-loss-health-changes

Bradley, S., & Miller, K. (2021, January 15). *These Intermittent Fasting Apps Make It *So* Simple To Stay On Track*. Women's Health.

https://www.womenshealthmag.com/weight-loss/g29554400/inter-mittent-fasting-apps/

Bray, K. (2015, March 13). *Fasting diets may affect medication - Medicines and supplements.* CHOICE. https://www.choice.com.au/health-and-body/medicines-and-supplements/prescription-medicines/articles/fasting-diets-and-medication-160315

Brennan, D. (2020, September 17). *Health Benefits of Potatoes.* WebMD. https://www.webmd.com/diet/health-benefits-potatoes#:~:text=Potatoes%20are%20a%20good%20source

Brennan, D. (2021, October 25). *Psychological Benefits of Fasting.* WebMD. https://www.webmd.com/diet/psychological-benefits-of-fasting

Brick, S. (2021, May 21). *Is Alternate-Day Fasting Really That Good for You? We Dig.* Greatist. https://greatist.com/health/alternate-day-fasting#fasting-day-foods-drinks

Brill, J. (2021, March 23). *The 16:8 Time-Restricted Intermittent Fasting Plan.* Dummies. https://www.dummies.com/article/body-mind-spirit/physical-health-well-being/diet-nutrition/intermittent-fasting/the-168-time-restricted-intermittent-fasting-plan-275811/

Brown, S. (n.d.). *Intermittent Fasting and Binge Eating: What The Research Shows.* Binge Eating Hope. https://www.bingeeatinghope.com/blog/intermittent-fasting

Bryan, L. (2021, July 4). *40+ Easy & Healthy Salad Recipes.* Downshiftology. https://downshiftology.com/salad-recipes/

Bubnis, D. (2018, October 26). *How to Exercise Safely During Intermittent Fasting.* Healthline. https://www.healthline.com/health/how-to-exercise-safely-intermittent-fasting#effective-workouts-while-fasting

Calabrese, E. (2021, January 19). *Healthy Seafood Recipes, From Air Fryer Fish to Seared Ahi Tuna.* Delish. https://www.delish.com/cooking/nutrition/g928/healthy-seafood-recipes-myplate/

Cameron, M. (2021, December 2). *15 Easy Frittata Recipes That Are Perfect for Weight Loss.* Eat This Not That. https://www.eatthis.com/healthy-frittata-recipes/

Chaix, A., Deota, S., Bhardwaj, R., Lin, T., & Panda, S. (2021). *Sex- and age-dependent outcomes of 9-hour time-restricted feeding of a Western high-fat high-sucrose diet in C57BL/6J mice.* Cell Reports, 36(7), 109543. https://doi.org/10.1016/j.celrep.2021.109543

Chan, T. (2021, January 4). *Does Taking Medication Break Intermittent Fasting?* Simple.life Blog. https://simple.life/blog/intermittent-fasting-and-medication/#:~:text=There%20are%20many%20ways%20that

Chicago, U. of I. at. (2022, January 1). *Research Shows Intermittent Fasting Works for Weight Loss.* SciTechDaily. https://scitechdaily.com/research-shows-intermittent-fasting-works-for-weight-loss/

Citroner, G. (2021, November 16). *Fasting for 24 Hours May Reduce Diabetes and Heart Disease Risk.* Healthline. https://www.healthline.com/health-news/intermittent-fasting-once-a-week-may-reduce-diabetes-and-heart-disease-risk#Inflammation-and-heart-health

Contributors, W. E. (2020, August 24). *Health Benefits of Beans.* WebMD. https://www.webmd.com/diet/health-benefits-beans

Control, I. (2018, June 9). *Prevent Diabetes With Intermittent Fasting? Diabetes in Control.* A Free Weekly Diabetes Newsletter for Medical Professionals.; Diabetes In Control. A free weekly diabetes newsletter for Medical Professionals. https://www.diabetesincontrol.com/prevent-diabetes-with-intermittent-fasting/

Cording, J. (2021, February 25). *Distracted At Work Because You're Fasting? Here's How To Refocus And Fuel Your Mind And Body.* Forbes. https://www.forbes.com/sites/jesscording/2021/02/25/distracted-at-work-because-youre-fasting--heres-how--to-refocus-and-fuel-your-mind-and-body/?sh=56e486ba7a4a

Corte, M. L., & Lobel, N. (2022, February 4). *73 Healthy Lunch Ideas You'll Actually Be Excited to Eat.* Delish. https://www.delish.com/cooking/nutrition/g1441/healthy-packed-lunches/

CTCA. (2021, June 9). *What you need to know about fasting and cancer.* Cancer Treatment Centers of America. https://www.cancercenter.com/community/blog/2021/06/fasting-cancer

Cunff, A.-L. L. (2020, August 12). *The mindful productivity guide to intermittent fasting.* Ness Labs. https://nesslabs.com/mindful-productivity-intermittent-fasting

DiCenso, B. (2021, November 25). *70+ Best Healthy Egg Recipes for Weight Loss.* Eat This%2c Not That! https://www.eatthis.com/healthy-egg-recipes/

Duck, mango and watercress salad. (2016, April 16). Www.olivemagazine.com. https://www.olivemagazine.com/recipes/meat-and-poultry/duck-mango-and-watercress-salad/

Elliott, M. (2017, July 18). *14 Healthy Snacks Made With Fruit to Eat This Week.* Showbiz Cheat Sheet. https://www.cheatsheet.com/culture/super-healthy-snacks-made-with-fruit.html/

Ellis, E. (2020, August 13). *The Beginners Guide to Cruciferous Vegetables.* Www.eatright.org. https://www.eatright.org/food/vitamins-and-supplements/nutrient-rich-foods/the-beginners-guide-to-cruciferous-vegetables#:~:text=Most%20cruciferous%20vegetables%20are%20rich

Fern, C. (2019, February 27). *These Cheese Snacks are So Insanely Good You'll Want to Skip Dinner.* Oprah Daily. https://www.oprahdaily.com/life/food/g26539733/best-cheese-snacks/

5 Ways to Stay Motivated when Doing Intermittent Fasting. (2021, July 28). BodyFast. https://www.bodyfast.app/en/motivation-for-intermittent-fasting/

Fletcher, J. (2019, April 5). *Intermittent fasting for weight loss: 5 tips to start.* Www.medicalnewstoday.com. https://www.medicalnewstoday.com/articles/324882#:~:text=The%20easiest%20way%20to%20do

Florio, G. (2018, June 26). *Stay Busy While You're Fasting.* POPSUGAR Fitness. https://www.popsugar.com/fitness/photo-gallery/44971477/image/44971536/Stay-Busy-While-Youre-Fasting

40+ Healthy Ground Beef Recipes. (2021, August 6). Jar of Lemons. https://www.jaroflemons.com/healthy-ground-beef-recipes/

Garrison, L. (2021). *Intermittent Fasting Can Aid in Weight Loss, Anti-Aging, and Overall Health.* Bizjournals.com. https://www.bizjournals.com/twincities/news/2020/02/28/intermittent-fasting-can-aid-in-weight-loss-anti.html

Gogos, D. K. (2015, March 10). *The history of fasting.* NEOS KOSMOS. https://neoskosmos.com/en/2015/03/10/life/food-drink/the-history-of-fasting/

A Guide To The 20:4 Fast. (2020). MealPrep. https://www.mealprep.com.au/intermittent-fasting/a-guide-to-the-204-fast/

Gunnars, K. (2017, June 4). *What Is Intermittent Fasting? Explained in Human Terms.* Healthline. https://www.healthline.com/nutrition/what-is-intermittent-fasting#TOC_TITLE_HDR_2

Gunnars, K. (2018, June 28). *Top 10 Health Benefits of Eating Eggs.* Healthline. https://www.healthline.com/nutrition/10-proven-health-benefits-of-eggs#TOC_TITLE_HDR_6

Gunnars, K. (2020, September 25). *How Intermittent Fasting Can Help You Lose Weight.* Healthline. https://www.healthline.com/nutrition/intermittent-fasting-and-weight-loss#weight-loss

Haney, S. (2022, January 31). *This Is How Long It'll Take For Intermittent Fasting to Work.* POPSUGAR Fitness. https://www.popsugar.com/fitness/How-Long-Does-Take-Intermittent-Fasting-Work-45006826

Hanka, S. (2021, July 17). *How to Intermittent Fast: 6 Tips to Get Started.* Www.trifectanutrition.com. https://www.trifectanutrition.-com/blog/how-to-intermittent-fast-6-tips-to-get-started

Health Benefits of Fish | DOH. (n.d.). Doh.wa.gov. https://doh.wa.-gov/community-and-environment/food/fish/health-bene-fits#:~:text=Fish%20is%20filled%20with%20omega

Hill, A. (2020, January 7). *Eat Stop Eat Review: Does It Work for Weight Loss?* Healthline. https://www.healthline.com/nutrition/eat-stop-eat-review#the-diet

Hilton, C., ersen, & Karasik, C. S. (2021, July 20). *These Protein-Packed Healthy Breakfasts Will Make Losing Weight So Much Easier.* Women's Health. https://www.womenshealthmag.com/weight-loss/a19993913/protein-breakfast-ideas/

Hindy, J. (2014, August 20). *15 Amazing Health Benefits Of Berries You Didn't Know About.* Lifehack. https://www.lifehack.org/articles/life-style/15-amazing-health-benefits-berries-you-didnt-know-about.html

Hopkins, J. (2022). *Intermittent Fasting: What is it, and how does it work?* Www.hopkinsmedicine.org. https://www.hopkinsmedi-cine.org/health/wellness-and-prevention/intermittent-fasting-what-is-it-and-how-does-it-work#:~:text=What%20is%20intermittent%20-fasting%3F

Horton, B. (2019, April 2). *You're Probably Doing Intermittent Fasting the Wrong Way—Here's Why.* Cooking Light. https://www.cookinglight.-com/eating-smart/nutrition-101/intermittent-fasting-mistakes

How to Break a Fast. (2022, January 10). WikiHow. https://www.wiki-how.com/Break-a-Fast

Intermittent Fasting and Hydration: Complete Guide (Updated 2022). (n.d.). Copper H2O. Retrieved April 23, 2022, from https://www.cop-perh2o.com/blogs/blog/the-complete-guide-to-intermittent-fasting-

and-proper-
hydration#:~:text=Some%20of%20the%20symptoms%20of

Intermittent Fasting May Help Cancer Treatments Work Better, Small, Early Study Suggests. (2021, November 30). Www.breastcancer.org. https://www.breastcancer.org/research-news/intermittent-fasting-may-help-cancer-treatments-work-better

I. T. W. D.(2016, October 19). *The Right Way to Break the Fast: What to eat when.* India Today. https://www.indiatoday.in/lifestyle/well-ness/story/right-way-to-break-the-fast-starvation-karva-chauth-enzymes-fasting-lifest-347386-2016-10-19

Jarreau, P. (2019a, February 26). *The 5 stages of intermittent fasting.* LIFE Apps | LIVE and LEARN. https://lifeapps.io/fasting/the-5-stages-of-intermittent-fasting/

Jarreau, P. (2019b, June 11). *It's Time to Recycle... Your Cells. Daily Fasting Activates Autophagy.* LIFE Apps | LIVE and LEARN. https://lifeapps.io/fasting/its-time-to-recycle-your-cells-daily-fast-ing-activates-autophagy/

Jennings, K.-A. (2016). *9 Legitimate Health Benefits of Eating Whole Grains.* Healthline. https://www.healthline.com/nutrition/9-benefits-of-whole-grains

Johnson, J. (2019, January 28). *The 5:2 diet: A guide and meal plan.* Www.medicalnewstoday.com. https://www.medicalnewstoday.-com/articles/324303#what-is-the-52-diet

Johnson, O. (2021, March 24). *Best Foods To Break A Fast: Top 14 Foods That Make The Fast To Feast Transition Smooth.* BetterMe Blog. https://betterme.world/articles/best-foods-to-break-a-fast/

Kabala, J. (2018). *The Top 9 Nuts to Eat for Better Health.* Healthline. https://www.healthline.com/nutrition/9-healthy-nuts

Karima, H. (2021, April 18). *5 Tips to Stay More Focused and Productive at Work While Fasting.* EgyptToday. https://www.egypttoday.com/Article/6/101012/5-Tips-to-Stay-More-Focused-and-Productive-at-Work

Kaupe, A. (2019, March 8). *How to do Intermittent Fasting According to 40 Famous People.* 21 Day Hero. https://21dayhero.com/how-to-do-intermittent-fasting-according-to-famous-people/#:~:text=Actresses%20Nicole%20Kidman%20and%20Halle

Kay, S. (2021). *High-Protein Breakfast Foods.* Kaynutrition.com. https://kaynutrition.com/9-high-protein-breakfast-foods/

Kim. (2021, January 12). *25 High Protein Lunch Ideas (+ Easy Recipes).* Insanely Good Recipes. https://insanelygoodrecipes.com/high-protein-lunch-ideas/

Kubala, J. (2018, July 3). *The Warrior Diet: Review and Beginner's Guide.* Healthline. https://www.healthline.com/nutrition/warrior-diet-guide#how-to-follow

Landau, D. (2022, January 21). *Intermittent Fasting and Rheumatoid Arthritis: What to Know.* EverydayHealth.com. https://www.everyday-health.com/rheumatoid-arthritis/things-people-with-rheumatoid-arthritis-should-know-about-intermittent-fasting/

Langness, D. (2019, March 3). *When and Why Did Humans Start Fasting?* Bahaiteachings.org/. https://bahaiteachings.org/when-why-did-humans-start-fasting/

Lederer, S. (2020, October 13). *How to Break a Fast: 10 Best Foods (Intermittent & Prolonged).* Mental Food Chain. https://www.mentalfood-chain.com/break-a-fast/

Leech, J. (2019, June 11). *11 Evidence-Based Health Benefits of Eating Fish.* Healthline. https://www.healthline.com/nutrition/11-health-benefits-of-fish#TOC_TITLE_HDR_3

Leonard, J. (2020, April 16). *Seven ways to do intermittent fasting: The best methods.* Www.medicalnewstoday.com. https://www.medicalnew-stoday.com/articles/322293#:~:text=The%20easiest%20way%20to%20do

Lewin, J. (2019). *The Health Benefits Of Eggs.* BBC Good Food. https://www.bbcgoodfood.com/howto/guide/ingredient-focus-eggs

Link, R. (2021, March 22). *Drinking Water While Fasting: Is It Recommended?* Healthline. https://www.healthline.com/nutrition/can-you-drink-water-when-fasting#drinks-to-avoid

Livermore, S. (2018, August 13). *36 Healthier Ways To Cook Beef Your Diet Needs.* Delish. https://www.delish.com/cooking/g3789/healthy-beef-recipes/

Livermore, S., & Villarosa, D. (2021, September 3). *30 Healthy Ground Turkey Recipes That'll Make You Forget About Beef.* Delish. https://www.delish.com/cooking/g3765/healthy-ground-turkey-recipes/

Livermore, S., & Villarosa, D. (2022, February 26). *75 Chicken Recipes So Good You Won't Even Realize They're Healthy.* Delish. https://www.delish.com/cooking/g3456/healthy-chicken-recipes/

Long, K. (2021, November 18). *Intermittent Fasting May Protect the Heart by Controlling Inflammation.* Www.heart.org. https://www.heart.org/en/news/2021/11/18/intermittent-fasting-may-protect-the-heart-by-controlling-inflammation

Maldonado, J. (2022, March 11). *43 Healthy and Easy to Make Seafood Recipes.* Eat This Not That. https://www.eatthis.com/healthy-easy-seafood-recipes/

Manager, C. (n.d.). *How to Choose an Intermittent Fasting Schedule.* Carb Manager. https://www.carbmanager.com/article/yoherxeaaceaza-yu/how-to-choose-an-intermittent-fasting-schedule/

Marshall, C. (2021, October 14). *26 Easy High Protein Breakfast Recipes.* The Kitchen Community. https://thekitchencommunity.org/high-protein-breakfast-recipes/

McAuliffe, L. (2022, January 3). *The 20 Hour Fast: Benefits and How To*. Dr. Robert Kiltz. https://www.doctorkiltz.com/20-hour-fast/#:~:text=The%2020%20hour%20fast%20is

McKeehan, N. (2016). *Can Intermittent Fasting Help Prevent Dementia?* | Cognitive Vitality | Alzheimer's Drug Discovery Foundation. Alzdiscovery.org. https://www.alzdiscovery.org/cognitive-vitali-ty/blog/can-intermittent-fasting-help-prevent-dementia#:~:text=While%20these%20studies%20are%20promising

Midland, N. (2020, June 26). *Intermittent Fasting 14/10: A Step-By-Step Strategy To Knock Off Those Unwanted Pounds*. BetterMe Blog. https://betterme.world/articles/intermittent-fasting-14-10/

Miller, K. (2021, March 1). *The Eat Stop Eat Diet Involves Fasting For 24 Hours At A Time*. Women's Health. https://www.womenshealthmag.-com/weight-loss/a22689488/eat-stop-eat-diet/

MS, A. B., CCN. (2021, January 27). *Does Sleeping Count As Fasting? [Intermittent Fasting Tips]*. AutumnElleNutrition. https://www.autum-nellenutrition.com/post/does-sleeping-count-as-fasting

Najafi, C. (2015, June 14). *Fruit Breakfast Bowl Recipe*. Everyday Dishes. https://everydaydishes.com/simple-food-recipes/fruit-breakfast-bowl/

Nast, C. (2018, February 5). *19 Healthy Frittata Recipes That Are Perfect for Meal Prep*. SELF. https://www.self.com/gallery/frittata-recipes

National MS Society. (2018, July 12). *Intermittent Fasting Changes Gut Bacteria and Reduces MS-Like Symptoms in Mice*. National Multiple Sclerosis Society; National MS Society. https://www.nationalmssoci-ety.org/About-the-Society/News/Intermittent-Fasting-Changes-Gut-Bacteria-and-Redu

9 Intermittent Fasting Mistakes (And How To Avoid Them!). (2020, April 18). A Sweet Pea Chef. https://www.asweetpeachef.com/intermittent-fasting-mistakes/

Nutra, D. (2021, December 19). *Apple Cider Vinegar & Intermittent Fasting: Will ACV Break a Fast?* Divinity Nutra. https://divinitynutra.com/health/apple-cider-vinegar-fasting/#:~:text=No%2C%20drinking%20apple%20cider%20vinegar%20will%20not%20break%20a%20fast.&text=Its%20overall%20calorie%20intake%20also

Orlov, A. (2022, January 4). 5 Free Meal Planning Templates to Simplify Your Life. Life by Daily Burn. https://dailyburn.com/life/health/printable-meal-planning-templates/

Petrucci, K., & Flynn, P. (2016, March 27). *10 Ways to Stay Motivated When Fasting.* Dummies. https://www.dummies.com/article/body-mind-spirit/physical-health-well-being/diet-nutrition/general-diet-nutrition/10-ways-to-stay-motivated-when-fasting-203870/

Phillips, H. (2020, April 1). *Feeling Nauseous While Intermittent Fasting?* Here's Why an RD Wants You to Take Caution. Sports.yahoo.com. https://sports.yahoo.com/feeling-nauseous-while-intermittent-fasting-002231872.html#:~:text=Your%20body%20needs%20time%20to

Pire, T., & 2021. (2021, June 2). *34 High-Protein Lunches That Are Simple, Satisfying and Scrumptious.* PureWow. https://www.purewow.com/food/high-protein-lunches

Prakash, S. (2021, August 25). *45 Easy Dinners That Are Mostly Vegetables.* Kitchn. https://www.thekitchn.com/10-dinners-that-are-mostly-vegetables-250208

Pridgett, T. (2021, December 16). *I Tried 12-Hour Fasting For 21 Days — Here Are the 3 Major Changes That Happened to My Body.* POPSUGAR Fitness. https://www.popsugar.com/fitness/What-1212-Fasting-45319996#:~:text=12%3A12%20is%20a%20type

Raman, R. (2018, March 14). *7 Health and Nutrition Benefits of Potatoes.* Healthline. https://www.healthline.com/nutrition/benefits-of-potatoes#TOC_TITLE_HDR_7

Rizzo, N., MS, & RD. (2021, June 14). *Celebrities Swear by the 5:2 Intermittent Fasting Diet to Lose Weight.* Men's Health. https://www.menshealth.com/nutrition/a36716421/5-2-diet-plan/

Robinson, J. (2013, April 2). *Eat, Fast And Live Longer With Michael Mosley.* KPBS Public Media. https://www.kpbs.org/news/arts-culture/2013/04/02/eat-fast-and-live-longer-michael-mosley

Roizen, M. (2022). *Why should I listen to my body when doing intermittent fasting (IF)?* | Dieting For Weight Loss. Sharecare. https://www.sharecare.com/health/dieting-for-weight-loss/why-listen-body-intermittent-fasting

Rosen, C. (2020, August 8). *30 Easy Seafood Recipes.* A Couple Cooks. https://www.acouplecooks.com/easy-seafood-recipes/

Ryan, T. (2021, June 3). *The Benefits of Intermittent Fasting for Sleep.* Sleep Foundation. https://www.sleepfoundation.org/physical-health/intermittent-fasting-sleep

Schenkman, L. (2020, July 20). *The science behind intermittent fasting — and how you can make it work for you.* Ideas.ted.com. https://ideas.ted.com/the-science-behind-intermittent-fasting-and-how-you-can-make-it-work-for-you/

Scher, B. (2021, March 21). *Intermittent Fasting: How to Break Your Fast.* Diet Doctor. https://www.dietdoctor.com/intermittent-fasting/how-to-break-your-fast#:~:text=Avoid%20breaking%20your%20fast%20with

17 Cheese Snacks We Can't Resist. (2021, August 3). Insanely Good Recipes. https://insanelygoodrecipes.com/cheese-snacks/

Shoemaker, S. (2021, April 7). *Does Apple Cider Vinegar Break a Fast?* Healthline. https://www.healthline.com/nutrition/does-apple-cider-vinegar-break-a-fast

Smith, J. (2017, December 31). *I Replaced Bone Broth for Breakfast to See If It Truly Curbs Hunger.* Brit + Co. https://www.brit.co/living/healthy-eating/bone-broth-for-breakfast/

Smith, J., & Risher, B. (2021, March 11). *These Delicious High-Protein Breakfast Ideas Will Keep You Going All Day Long.* Prevention. https://www.prevention.com/food-nutrition/healthy-eating/g23709836/high-protein-breakfasts/

Spritzler, F. (2019, January 17). *8 Health Benefits of Eating Nuts.* Health-line. https://www.healthline.com/nutrition/8-benefits-of-nuts#TOC_TITLE_HDR_2

Stanko, C. (2022, February 25). *60 Healthy Seafood Recipes.* Taste of Home. https://www.tasteofhome.com/collection/healthy-seafood-recipes/

Stice, E., Davis, K., Miller, N. P., & Marti, C. N. (2008). *Fasting Increases Risk for Onset of Binge Eating and Bulimic Pathology: A 5-Year Prospective Study.* Journal of Abnormal Psychology, 117(4), 941–946. https://doi.org/10.1037/a0013644

Stieg, C. (2020, January 15). *Twitter CEO Jack Dorsey: "I eat seven meals every week, just dinner."* CNBC. https://www.cnbc.com/2020/01/15/twitter-ceo-jack-dorsey-eats-seven-meals-every-week-only-dinner.html

Stiehl, C. (2018, November 23). *How Many Calories Can I Eat on Intermittent Fasting?* | POPSUGAR Fitness. POPSUGAR Fitness. https://www.popsugar.com/fitness/How-Many-Calories-Can-I-Eat-Intermittent-Fasting-45473251

Streit, L. (2019, September 6). *25 Easy Vegetable Snacks for Work and School.* It's a Veg World after All®. https://itsavegworldafterall.com/25-easy-vegetable-snacks/

Strong, J., & McClintock, J. (1880). *Fasting in the Christian Church from the McClintock and Strong Biblical Cyclopedia.* McClintock and Strong Biblical Cyclopedia Online. https://www.biblicalcyclopedia.com/F/fasting-in-the-christian-church.html

Suazo, A. (2021, February 18). *Types of Fasting Diets and How to Choose the Right One.* Bulletproof. https://www.bulletproof.com/diet/intermittent-fasting/fasting-diet-types/

Talmadge, C. (2021, October 27). *37+ Best Healthy Ground Beef Recipes for Weight Loss.* Eat This Not That. https://www.eatthis.com/healthy-ground-beef-recipes/

Tarlton, Amanda. (2022, January 5). *50 Healthy Beef Dinners.* Taste of Home. https://www.tasteofhome.com/collection/healthy-beef-dinners/

Tello, M. (2018, June 26). *Intermittent Fasting: Surprising Update - Harvard Health Blog.* Harvard Health Blog. https://www.health.harvard.edu/blog/intermittent-fasting-surprising-update-2018062914156

These 5 Healthy Yogurt Parfaits are Perfect for Meal Prepping as a Breakfast, Snack or Even Dessert! Made with Protein Packed Yogurt + Easily Customizable! (2019, January 13). The Clean Eating Couple. https://thecleaneatingcouple.com/5-healthy-yogurt-parfaits/

13 Healthy Omelette Recipes | Popular Egg Recipes. (2022). NDTV Food. https://food.ndtv.com/lists/10-best-omelette-recipes-774333

37 Best Salad Recipes. (2019, July 1). Love and Lemons. https://www.loveandlemons.com/salad-recipes/

36 Must-Make Cheese Appetizers For People Who Love Party Food. (n.d.). Cooper Cheese. Retrieved April 23, 2022, from https://www.coopercheese.com/recipe/cheese-appetizers/

Time to try intermittent fasting? (2020, July 1). Harvard Health. https://www.health.harvard.edu/heart-health/time-to-try-intermittent-fasting#:~:text=Keto%20is%20short%20for%20ketosis

Tinsley, G. (2017, September 17). *Time-Restricted Eating: A Beginner's Guide.* Healthline. https://www.healthline.com/nutrition/time-restricted-eating#TOC_TITLE_HDR_5

Tropical Fruit Breakfast Parfaits. (2016, July 13). The Busy Baker. https://thebusybaker.ca/tropical-fruit-breakfast-parfaits/

Trumpfeller, G. (2020, March 20). *Autophagy and Intermittent Fasting - Is It Healthy?* Simple.life Blog. https://simple.life/blog/autophagy/

25 Nut Snack Recipes for Healthier Snacking. (2012, June 18). Snappy Living. https://snappyliving.com/25-nut-snack-recipes/

24 Healthy Veggie-Packed Dinners to Make During the Week. (2019, February 17). Ambitious Kitchen. https://www.ambitiouskitchen.com/healthy-veggie-packed-dinners/

Valente, L. (2021, July 7). *50+ Cheap Healthy Lunch Ideas for Work.* EatingWell. https://www.eatingwell.com/gallery/11785/cheap-healthy-lunch-ideas-for-work

Vigoreaux, G., & Lo, C. (2021, May 27). *37 Delicious Healthy Salads That Are Fresh and Filling.* Good Housekeeping. https://www.goodhousekeeping.com/food-recipes/healthy/g180/healthy-salads/

Villines, Z. (2020, January 16). *9 health benefits of beans.* Www.medical-newstoday.com. https://www.medicalnewstoday.com/articles/320192#benefits

Waterhouse, J. (2022). *9 Celebrities Who Swear By Intermittent Fasting.* Marie Claire. https://www.marieclaire.com.au/intermittent-fasting-celebrities

Watson, S. (2021, March 5). *Can Intermittent Fasting Help MS?* WebMD. https://www.webmd.com/multiple-sclerosis/multiple-sclerosis-intermittent-fasting

Weg, A. (2018, May 7). *15 Tasty, Uncomplicated High-Protein Lunches.* Cooking Light. https://www.cookinglight.com/food/quick-healthy/easy-high-protein-lunches

What Are Cruciferous Vegetables — and Why Are They So Good for You? (2020, December 9). Health Essentials from Cleveland Clinic.

https://health.clevelandclinic.org/crunchy-and-cruciferous-youll-love-this-special-family-of-veggies/

Working Out While Intermittent Fasting | Prospect Medical Systems. (2021). Www.prospectmedical.com. https://www.prospectmedical.com/resources/wellness-center/working-out-while-intermittent-fasting#:~:text=The%20best%20time%20to%20work

Yeager, S. (2019, May 16). *An Avocado-Rich Breakfast Can Help You Feel Fuller for Longer.* Bicycling. https://www.bicycling.com/health-nutrition/a27465835/avocado-breakfast-hunger-suppression/#:~:text=Avocados%20contain%20high%20amounts%20of

Yoon, G., & Song, J. (2019). *Intermittent Fasting: a Promising Approach for Preventing Vascular Dementia.* Journal of Lipid and Atherosclerosis, 8(1), 1–7. https://doi.org/10.12997/jla.2019.8.1.1

Yovino, K. (2015, June 10). *6 Healthy Nut Snack Recipes That Fill You Up, Not Make You Fat.* Showbiz Cheat Sheet. https://www.cheatsheet.com/life/6-healthy-snack-recipes-starring-nutrient-rich-nuts.html/

Yu, C., & Shacknai, G. (2021, July 19). *Switch Up Your Go-To Scramble With These Delicious Egg Breakfast Recipes.* Women's Health.

Zelman, K. M., MPH, RD, & LD. (2011, June 21). *Tips for Reaping the Benefits of Whole Grains.* WebMD. https://www.webmd.com/food-recipes/features/reap-the-benefits-of-whole-grains#:~:text=Whole%20grains%20are%20packed%20with

Zentrum fuer Diabetesforschung DZD, D. (2019, July 2). *Promising approach: Prevent diabetes with intermittent fasting.* ScienceDaily. https://www.sciencedaily.com/releases/2019/07/190702152749.htm

IMAGE REFERENCES

FoodieFactor. (2017, August 23). *Food Egg Eggs Toast Toasted Bread.* Pixabay.com.　https://pixabay.com/photos/food-egg-eggs-toast-toasted-bread-2673724/

HappyVeganFit. (2019, October 19). *Remove Weight Loss Slim Diet.* Pixabay.com. https://pixabay.com/photos/remove-weight-loss-slim-diet-4559326/

Pexels. (2016, March 27). *Arm Hand Write Planner Planning.* Pixabay.com. https://pixabay.com/photos/arm-hand-write-planner-planning-1284248/

Psychoconsultants. (2021, June 2). *Woman Adult Yoga Zen Meditate.* Pixabay.com. https://pixabay.com/photos/woman-adult-yoga-zen-meditate-6304184/

PublicDomainPictures. (2014, April 5) *Buffet Indian Food Spices Lunch.* Pixabay.com. https://pixabay.com/photos/buffet-indian-food-spices-lunch-315691/

RitaE. (2016). *Yogurt Berry Blueberries Desert.* Pixabay.com. https://pixabay.com/photos/yogurt-berry-blueberries-dessert-1612787/

Silviarita. (2017, August 12). *Dragon Woman Human Stone Pebble.* Pixabay.com. https://pixabay.com/photos/dragon-woman-human-stone-pebble-2634391/

Silviarita. (2020, January 27). *Food Snack Loaf Sandwich Brunch.* Pixabay.com. https://pixabay.com/photos/food-snack-loaf-sandwich-brunch-4794790/

Stenholz. (2015, September 22). *Vegan Wrap Herbal Meal Healthy.* Pixabay.com. https://pixabay.com/photos/vegan-wrap-herbal-meal-healthy-946034/

StockSnap. (2017, August 1). *White Window Glass Shield Frame.* Pixabay.com. https://pixabay.com/photos/white-window-glass-shield-frame-2563976/

PART II
BONUS RECIPES AND MEAL PLAN

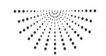

10

BREAKFAST RECIPES

Your morning sets up the success of your day... I use my first hour awake for my morning routine of breakfast and meditation to prepare myself. – Caroline Ghosn

Recipes in this chapter were selected as ideal candidates for the first meal after a fast. While they would work well with most of the IF methods, they are perfect for the time-restrictive methods 12:12, 16:8, and 18:6.

PROTEIN BERRY AND CARROT SMOOTHIE

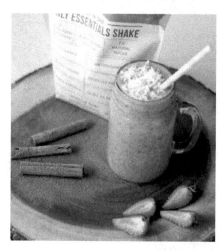

Per serving: 476 Calories • 72g Carbs (10.7g Fiber) • 9.7g Fat • 30.7g Protein

Ingredients scaled to: 1 serving

- 10 medium Baby carrots (100 grams)
- 2/3 Serving 100% Whey protein (66.7 grams)
- 1 medium (7" to 7-7/8" long) Banana (118 grams)
- 1/4 cup Blackberries (36 grams)
- 1/2 cup Blueberries (74 grams)
- 4 medium (1-1/4" dia) Strawberries (48 grams)
- 1 1/2 cups Reduced fat milk (366 grams)

Directions based on 1 serving

1. Combine all ingredients in a blender and pulse until smooth. Enjoy

STRAWBERRY YOGURT SMOOTHIE

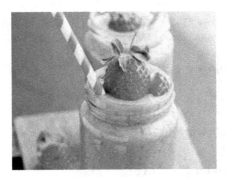

Per serving: 292 Calories • 21.7g Carbs (3g Fiber) • 16.5g Fat • 14.7g Protein

Ingredients scaled to: 1 serving

- 1 cup, halved Strawberries (152 grams)
- 1/2 cup Whole milk (122 grams)
- 1/2 cup Greek yogurt (120 grams)

Directions based on 1 serving

1. Combine all ingredients in a blender and pulse until smooth. Enjoy!

COTTAGE CHEESE & APPLESAUCE

Per serving: 214 Calories • 19.9g Carbs (1.4g Fiber) • 2.4g Fat • 28.2g Protein

Ingredients scaled to: 1 serving

- 1/2 cup Applesauce (61 grams)
- 1 cup Cottage cheese (113 grams)

Directions based on 1 serving

1. Mix together and enjoy!

SCRAMBLED EGGS WITH SPINACH AND CHEESE

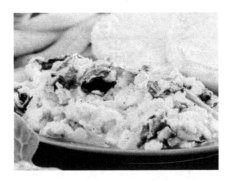

Per serving: 249 Calories • 2.8g Carbs (0.7g Fiber) • 17.4g Fat • 20.4g Protein

Ingredients scaled to: 1 serving

- 1/2 tsp Olive oil (2.3 grams)
- 1 cup Spinach (30 grams)
- 2 large Eggs (100 grams)
- 1/4 cup shredded Mexican cheese (28.3 grams)

Directions based on 1 serving

1. Heat a non-stick skillet over medium heat.
2. Coat spinach with olive oil and cook until slightly wilted, 3-4 minutes.
3. Reduce heat to medium-low.
4. Beat the eggs and add to the skillet with the spinach. Stir slowly over the heat until they reach your desired doneness. Sprinkle in the cheese and stir to combine and soften the cheese. Once cheese has melted, move the eggs to a plate and enjoy!

PEANUT BUTTER BANANA ENGLISH MUFFIN

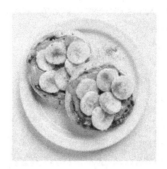

Per serving: 285 Calories • 44.8g Carbs (7.5g Fiber) • 9.8g Fat • 10.1g Protein

Ingredients scaled to: 1 serving

- 1 English muffin (66 grams)
- 1 tbsp Peanut butter (16 grams)
- 1/2 medium (7" to 7-7/8" long) Banana (59 grams)
- 1/2 tsp Cinnamon (1.3 grams)

DIRECTIONS BASED ON 1 SERVING

1. Toast the English muffin.
2. Top both sides of the English muffin with peanut butter, banana and cinnamon.

KETO BREAKFAST TACOS

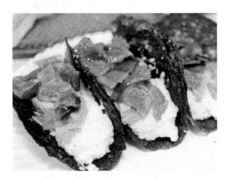

Per serving: 466 Calories • 5.5g Carbs (2.4g Fiber) • 37.1g Fat • 27.9g Protein

Ingredients scaled to: 3 servings

- 3 strips Bacon (36 grams)
- 1 cup diced Mozzarella cheese (132 grams)
- 6 large Eggs (300 grams)
- 2 tbsp Butter (28.4 grams)
- 1 tsp Salt (6 grams)
- 1 tsp Pepper (2.1 grams)
- 1/2 Avocado (101 grams)
- 1 oz Shredded Cheddar cheese (28.4 grams)

Directions based on 3 servings

1. Preheat the oven to 375°F.
2. Start off by cooking the bacon. Line a baking sheet with foil and bake 3 strips in an oven for about 15-20 minutes.
3. While the bacon is cooking, heat 1/3 cup of mozzarella in a clean pan on medium heat. This cheese will form our taco shells.
4. Wait until the cheese is browned on the edges (about 2-3 minutes). Slide a spatula under it to unstick it. This should

happen easily if you're using whole milk mozzarella as the oil from the cheese will prevent it from sticking.

5. Use a pair of tongs to lift the mozzarella cheese shell up and drape it over a wooden spoon that you have resting on a pot. Do the same with the rest of your cheese, working in batches of 1/3 cup.

6. Next, cook your eggs in the butter, season with salt and pepper while stirring occasionally until they're done..

7. Spoon a third of your scrambled eggs into each hardened taco shell.

8. Follow this by adding the bacon (either chopped or whole strips).

9. Lastly, sprinkle cheddar cheese over the tops of the breakfast tacos. Enjoy!

SPINACH AND SAUSAGE BREAKFAST MUFFIN

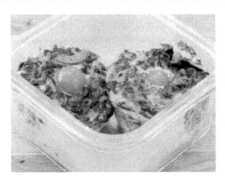

Per serving (one muffin): 164 Calories • 2.7g Carbs (0.5g Fiber) • 12.6g Fat • 9.8g Protein

Ingredients scaled to: 20 servings

- 2 1/2 cups fresh Spinach (75 grams)
- 16 oz Pork sausage (Without casing) (454 grams)
- 1 medium (approx 2-3/4" long, 2-1/2 dia.) Red bell pepper (Chopped) (119 grams)
- 1 cup, chopped Onion (160 grams)
- 8 oz Cheddar cheese (227 grams)
- 10 large Eggs (500 grams)
- 1/3 cup Heavy whipping cream (40 grams)
- 1 tbsp Onion powder (6.9 grams)
- 1 tbsp Garlic powder (9.7 grams)
- 1 tsp Salt (6 grams)
- 1 tbsp, ground Pepper (7.1 grams)

Directions based on 20 servings

1. Preheat the oven to 350 degrees °F.
2. Brown 16 oz of pork sausage in a skillet over medium heat until cooked through; add to a large bowl. Wipe the skillet clean.

3. Chop bell pepper and onion and add to the pan. Cook over medium heat for about 5-7 minutes, until onions are translucent then add the spinach until slightly wilted, add to the bowl with the sausage.
4. Add cheese to the bowl and mix together.
5. In a separate bowl whisk 10 eggs, cream, and spices. Add eggs to the rest of the ingredients and mix.
6. Split into 20 muffin cups.
7. Bake for 30 minutes or until a toothpick comes out clean.

KALE AND EGG CUPS

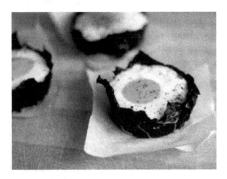

Per serving (two cups): 236 Calories • 7.9g Carbs (1.5g Fiber) • 15.7g Fat • 16.4g Protein

Ingredients scaled to: 2 servings

- 2 tsp Olive oil (9 grams)
- 6 oz Kale (4 large kale leaves, washed & trimmed) (170 grams)
- 4 extra-large Eggs (224 grams)
- 1 dash Salt (To taste) (0.40 grams)
- 1 dash Pepper (To taste) (0.10 grams)

Directions based on 2 servings

1. Preheat the oven to 375°F and grease a muffin tin with olive oil. Set aside.
2. In a large pot, bring approximately 4 cups of water to a boil. Add the kale leaves and cook for about 1 minute. Have a large bowl of ice water standing by.
3. When the Kale leaves have turned bright green and soft, remove from boiling water and immerse the leaves in the cold water to stop the cooking process.
4. Remove the cooled leaves from the ice water and pat dry with a paper towel. Line each cup of the muffin tin with a large kale leaf (trimming the edges if necessary).

5. Into each kale-lined cup, crack one egg. Sprinkle each with salt and pepper and bake for 20 minutes or until the egg is set.
6. Remove each egg cup from the muffin tin and serve warm.

OATMEAL AND APPLES

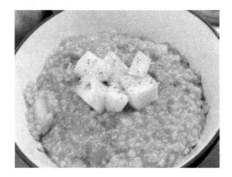

Per serving (one bowl): 270 Calories • 57.3g Carbs (11.1g Fiber) • 3.9g Fat • 6.5g Protein

Ingredients scaled to: 1 bowl

- 1/2 cup Oatmeal (40 grams)
- 1 tsp brown sugar (3.2 grams)
- 1 medium (3" dia) Apple (182 grams)
- 1 cup Pure Almond Milk (240 grams)

Directions based on 1 bowl

1. Peel the apple, remove the apple core and cut into slices. Mix together with almond milk and oats.
2. Microwave for 45 seconds, stir, then microwave for 30 more seconds. Sprinkle it with brown sugar and eat.

AVOCADO AND EGG TOAST

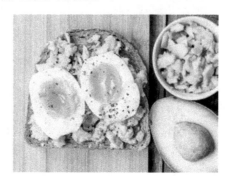

Per serving: 442 Calories • 31.9g Carbs (10.6g Fiber) • 26.4g Fat • 21.5g Protein

Ingredients scaled to: 1 serving

- 2 large Eggs (100 grams)
- 1/2 Avocado (101 grams)
- 2 slices of regular multi-grain bread (52 grams)

Directions based on 1 serving

1. Toast bread. Prepare egg as desired in a non-stick pan over medium heat.
2. Mash avocado.
3. Top toasted bread with the avocado mash. Finish with egg and enjoy!

11

LUNCH RECIPES

Ask not what you can do for your country. Ask what's for lunch. –Orson Wells

These recipes would go best with the time-restrictive IF methods: 12:12, 14:10, and 16:8.

TURKEY SALAD

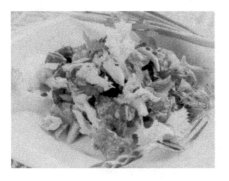

Per serving: 276 Calories • 4.1g Carbs (1g Fiber) • 9.5g Fat • 41.7g Protein

Ingredients scaled to: 1 serving

- 1 cup, chopped or diced Turkey, dark meat (5 oz) (142 grams)
- 1 cup shredded Lettuce (47 grams)
- 1 tbsp Mayonnaise-like dressing (14.7 grams)
- 1 serving Table Blend Salt Free Seasoning Blend (teaspoon) (1 grams)
- 1 dash Salt (0.40 grams)
- 1 dash Pepper (0.10 grams)
- 1 tsp Lemon juice (5.1 grams)

Directions based on 1 serving

1. Put seasonings, lemon juice, turkey, and mayo in a bowl. Mix well. Serve on top of lettuce.

CHICKEN LETTUCE WRAPS

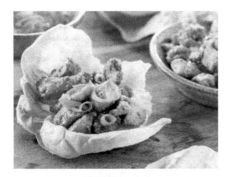

Per serving: 323 Calories • 4.1g Carbs (1g Fiber) • 18.2g Fat • 34.4g Protein

Ingredients scaled to: 1 serving

- 1/2 Chicken breast, bone and skin removed (Chopped) (118 grams)
- 1 tbsp Olive oil (13.5 grams)
- 1/4 cup chopped Onion (17.8 grams)
- 1/4 cup Cottage cheese (56.5 grams)
- 1 leaf of Butter Lettuce (15 grams)
- 1 tbsp Dijon mustard (15 grams)

Directions based on 1 serving

1. Chop chicken. Heat oil in a pan over medium-high heat and add chicken to the pan. Cook for 8-12 minutes until chicken is cooked through and no longer pink. Remove from heat and set aside.
2. Chop green onions and combine with chicken and cottage cheese. Scoop into lettuce leaves, season with a little dijon, wrap and serve.
3. Enjoy!

SPINACH, LEMON, AND SHRIMP SALAD

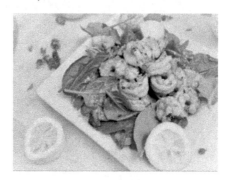

Per serving: 115 Calories • 3.1g Carbs (1.3g Fiber) • 5.6g Fat • 13.3g Protein

Ingredients scaled to: 2 servings

- 4 cups of Spinach (120 grams)
- 1 tsp Lemon juice (5.1 grams)
- 2 tsp Olive oil (9 grams)
- 6 oz peeled and deveined Shrimp (170 grams)

Directions based on 2 servings

1. Cook shrimp in boiling water until pink and opaque (done). Remove shells if present. Set shrimp on paper towels to dry.
2. Whisk lemon juice and olive oil together. Toss spinach leaves and shrimp in this dressing and enjoy!

CHICKEN, SPINACH, AND STRAWBERRY SALAD

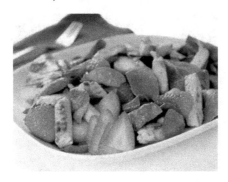

Per serving: 255 Calories • 11.7g Carbs (3.3g Fiber) • 10.3g Fat • 29.1g Protein

Ingredients scaled to: 2 servings

- 1 Chicken breast, bone and skin removed (236 grams)
- 4 cups Spinach (120 grams)
- 1 cup Strawberry halves (152 grams)
- 2/3 small raw Red Onion (thinly sliced) (46.6 grams)
- 1 tbsp Balsamic vinegar (16 grams)
- 1 tbsp Olive oil (13.5 grams)

Directions based on 2 servings

1. Preheat the oven to 400°F. Bake chicken for 10-15 minutes or until cooked through and no longer pink. Let rest for 5 minutes before slicing.
2. Combine all ingredients in a bowl and drizzle with salad dressing!
3. Enjoy!

FLANK STEAK AND TOMATOES

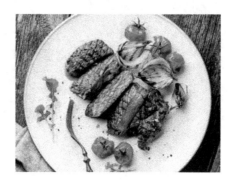

Per serving: 195 Calories • 1.7g Carbs (0.5g Fiber) • 9.4g Fat • 24.7g Protein

Ingredients scaled to: 4 servings

- 1 1/4 tsp ground Cumin (3 grams)
- 1 dash Salt (0.40 grams)
- 1 pinch Cayenne pepper (0.36 grams)
- Cooking spray (0.30 grams)
- 16 oz Beef flank (Trimmed of fat) (454 grams)
- 1 tbsp Olive oil (13.5 grams)
- 1 tsp chopped Garlic (5 grams)
- 1 jalapeño pepper (Chopped) (14 grams)
- 1/2 cup cherry tomatoes (74.5 grams)
- 1/4 cup Fresh cilantro (4 grams)

Directions based on 4 servings

1. Preheat the broiler to high.
2. In a small dish combine 1 teaspoon cumin, 1⁄2 teaspoon salt, and cayenne pepper, and sprinkle it over the steak.
3. Spray a broiler pan with cooking spray, then place the trimmed flank steak with seasoning in the pan to broil for about 10 minutes. Turn once and make sure it is cooked to the

proper doneness. Let rest 5 minutes before cutting the steak diagonally across the grain into thin slices.

4. While the steak is cooking, take a large nonstick skillet and heat oil over medium heat. Add the garlic and jalapeño into the pan and allow to cook for 1 minute. Then toss the remaining 1/4 teaspoon of cumin and salt along with the tomatoes into the pan. Allow the tomatoes to soften for 3 minutes, remove them from the heat and stir in the cilantro. Serve with the steak and enjoy!

BBQ CHICKEN SALAD

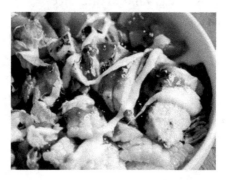

Per serving: 258 Calories • 21.8g Carbs (3.9g Fiber) • 6.7g Fat • 29.3g Protein

Ingredients scaled to: 2 servings

- 8 oz boneless skinless Chicken breast (227 grams)
- 1/2 tbsp Poultry seasoning (2.2 grams)
- Cooking spray (0.30 grams)
- 1 ear of corn, medium (6-3/4" to 7-1/2" long) (103 grams)
- 2 cups of shredded Lettuce (94 grams)
- 2 medium Tomatoes cut into quarters (2-3/5" diameter) (246 grams)
- 2 tbsp Sour cream (24 grams)
- 1 tbsp Ray's No Sugar Barbecue sauce (17.5 grams)

Directions based on 2 servings

1. Season the chicken with the poultry seasoning mix. Cook chicken on a grill or grill pan sprayed with oil over medium heat for about 5 minutes on each side, or until the chicken is cooked through in the center. Transfer to a cutting board, let it rest 5 minutes and slice thin.

2. Place the corn in the microwave for 4 minutes (or you can peel and boil in water for 5 minutes). Peel the husk off the corn, then cut the corn off the cob.
3. Divide the lettuce, tomatoes, corn, and chicken on two plates.
4. Combine the BBQ sauce with the sour cream and drizzle over the salad. Enjoy!

CHEESY BURGER STUFFED PORTOBELLOS

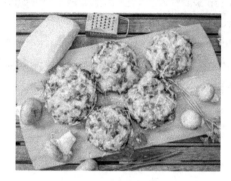

Per serving: 744 Calories • 5.3g Carbs (1.4g Fiber) • 63.4g Fat • 37.6g Protein

Ingredients scaled to: 2 servings

- 2 whole Portobello Mushrooms (168 grams)
- 10 oz Ground beef (284 grams)
- 4 oz Cheddar cheese (Grated) (113 grams)
- 1 cup Spinach (finely chopped) (30 grams)
- 2 tbsp Parmesan cheese (grated) (10 grams)
- 1 dash Salt (to taste) (0.40 grams)
- 1 dash Pepper (to taste) (0.10 grams)

Directions based on 2 servings

1. Preheat the oven to 375°F.
2. Remove the stems from the portobellos. Chop stems finely and add to the ground beef. With a spoon, scrape out the gills on the underside of the mushrooms and discard.
3. Finely chop spinach and grate cheese. Set aside.
4. Season the mushrooms with a sprinkling of salt and pepper. Mix the cheddar cheese and spinach into the ground beef. Season with a dash of salt and pepper. Form two patties and press them onto the portobello mushrooms.

5. Place the stuffed mushrooms on a small sheet pan or baking dish and cook for 20 minutes or until cooked through. Add the Parmesan cheese to the top of each and pop back into the oven to melt the cheese or under the broiler to brown. Serve hot and enjoy!

PALEO AVOCADO CHICKEN SALAD

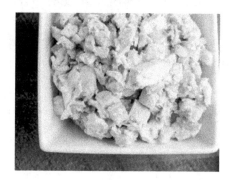

Per serving: 391 Calories • 17.6g Carbs (9.9g Fiber) • 24.2g Fat • 29.8g Protein

Ingredients scaled to: 1 serving

- 1 Avocado (136 grams)
- 1 Lemon juiced (47 grams)
- 1/4 medium (2-1/2" dia) Onion chopped (27.5 grams)
- 1 dash Salt (0.40 grams)
- 1 dash Pepper (0.10 grams)
- 1 cooked boneless skinless Chicken breast (86 grams)

Directions based on 1 serving

1. Cut the avocado in half and scoop the middle of both avocado halves into a bowl.
2. Add lemon juice and onion to the avocado in the bowl and mash together. Using two forks, shred chicken breast (or chop into chunks). Mix chicken, salt and pepper, and stir and add to the avocado mixture. Taste and adjust if needed. Serve and enjoy!

PALEO AVOCADO TUNA SALAD

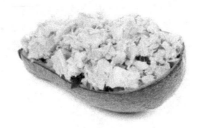

Per serving: 364 Calories • 16g Carbs (9.6g Fiber) • 22.4g Fat • 30.5g Protein

Ingredients scaled to: 1 serving

- 1 Avocado (136 grams)
- 1 Lemon juiced (47 grams)
- 1 tbsp chopped Onion (10 grams)
- 5 oz Tuna drained (142 grams)
- 1 dash Salt (0.40 grams)
- 1 dash Pepper (0.10 grams)

Directions based on 1 serving

1. Cut the avocado in half and scoop the middle of both avocado halves into a bowl, leaving a shell of avocado flesh about 1/4-inch thick on each half.
2. Add lemon juice and onion to the avocado in the bowl and mash together. Add drained tuna, salt and pepper, and stir to combine. Taste and adjust if needed.
3. Fill avocado shells with tuna salad and serve.

MEXICAN QUINOA

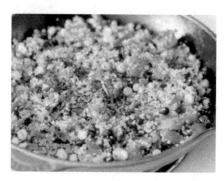

Per serving: 267 Calories • 46.1g Carbs (10.2g Fiber) • 5.3g Fat • 12.5g Protein

Ingredients scaled to: 4 servings

- 1 tbsp Olive oil (13.5 grams)
- 2 cloves, minced Garlic (6 grams)
- 1 cup Quinoa (170 grams)
- 1 1/2 cups Vegetable Broth (360 grams)
- 2 cups Black beans drained (388 grams)
- 1 3/4 cups chopped Tomatoes (422 grams)
- 1 cup kernels of Corn (164 grams)
- 1 tsp Chili powder (2.6 grams)
- 1/2 tsp, ground Cumin (1.5 grams)
- 1 dash Salt (0.40 grams)
- 1 dash Pepper (0.10 grams)
- Juice from 1 lime (44 grams)
- 1 tbsp Fresh cilantro (1 grams)

Directions based on 4 servings

1. Heat olive oil in a large skillet over medium high heat. Add garlic and cook, stirring frequently, until fragrant, about 1 minute.

2. Stir in quinoa, vegetable broth, beans, tomatoes, corn, chili powder, and cumin; season with salt and pepper, to taste. Bring to a boil; cover, reduce heat and simmer until quinoa is cooked through, about 20 minutes.
3. Stir in lime juice and cilantro. Serve immediately.

1 2
DINNER RECIPES

All great change in America begins at the dinner table. –Ronald Reagan

These recipes would work with all of the IF methods referenced in this book but would be of particular benefit to the longer fasts such as the 20:4, 5/2, Eat Stop Eat, and the Alternate Day Fasting methods.

MAPLE GLAZED CHICKEN

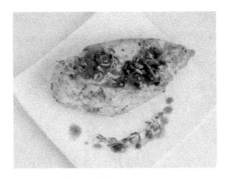

Per serving: 351 Calories • 10.6g Carbs (0.4g Fiber) • 8.9g Fat • 53.5g Protein

Ingredients scaled to: 2 servings

- 1 tbsp Maple syrup (20 grams)
- 1 tbsp Hoisin sauce (16 grams)
- 1 tsp Dijon mustard (5 grams)
- 1/4 tsp Pepper (0.53 grams)
- 1 tsp Vegetable oil (4.7 grams)
- 2 Chicken breasts, bone and skin removed (472 grams)

Directions based on 2 servings

1. Preheat the oven to 400°F.
2. Combine the first 4 ingredients in a small bowl; stir with a whisk.
3. Place chicken on a broiler pan coated with oil. Brush with maple mixture. Bake for 10 to 15 minutes, brushing with maple mixture after 5 minutes and again after 10 minutes. Cook until juices run clear and chicken is no longer pink, and the internal temperature is 165°F.
4. Pour the sauce (Step 2) over the chicken and serve. Enjoy!

PEPPERED STEAK WITH MUSHROOMS

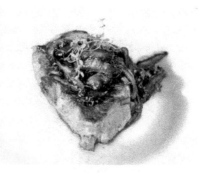

Per serving: 326 Calories • 2.8g Carbs (1g Fiber) • 24.2g Fat • 23.8g Protein

Ingredients scaled to: 4 servings

- 1 lb Beef tenderloin cut into 4 portions (454 grams)
- 1 tsp Pepper (2.1 grams)
- 1 tbsp Olive oil (13.5 grams)
- 1/4 cup Beef broth (60 grams)
- 3 cups diced Mushrooms (258 grams)

Directions based on 4 servings

1. Trim fat from steaks. Rub both sides of steaks with pepper. In a large skillet, heat olive oil over medium high heat.
2. Add steaks; reduce heat to medium. Cook to desired temperature, 7 to 9 minutes for medium rare (145°F) to medium (160°F), turning once halfway through cooking time.
3. Transfer steaks to a serving platter; keep warm.
4. Add beef broth to the skillet. Cook and stir until bubbly to loosen any browned bits in the bottom of the skillet. Add mushrooms; simmer, uncovered for 4 minutes. Spoon sauce over steaks to serve.

PHILLY CHEESESTEAK STUFFED HALVED PEPPERS

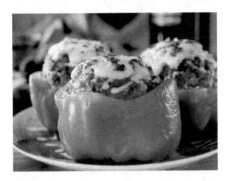

Per serving (one pepper): 442 Calories • 9.7g Carbs (2.4g Fiber) • 30.2g Fat • 33.7g Protein

Ingredients scaled to: 4 Peppers (4 servings)

- 8 oz Beef round (227 grams)
- 8 slices (1 oz) Provolone cheese (224 grams)
- 2 large Green bell peppers (2-1/4 per lb, approximately 3-3/4" long (328 grams)
- 1 medium Onion (2-1/2" dia) (110 grams)
- 1 1/2 cups, whole Mushrooms (144 grams)
- 2 tbsp Butter (28.4 grams)
- 2 tbsp Olive oil (27 grams)
- 1 tbsp Garlic (8.5 grams)

Directions based on 4 servings

1. Slice peppers in half lengthwise, remove ribs and seeds. Set aside.
2. Slice onions and mushrooms. Sauté over medium heat with butter, olive oil, minced garlic and a little salt and pepper. Sauté until onions and mushrooms are nice and caramelized. About 25-30 minutes.
3. Preheat the oven to 400°F.

4. Slice roast beef into thin strips and add to the onion/mushroom mixture. Allow to cook 5-10 minutes

5. Line the inside of each pepper with a slice of provolone cheese.

6. Fill each pepper with meat mixture until they are nearly overflowing. Top each pepper with another slice of provolone cheese.

7. Bake for 15-20 minutes until the cheese on top is golden brown.

SPINACH AND MUSHROOM SMOTHERED GRILLED CHICKEN

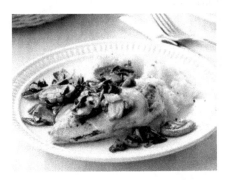

Per serving: 379 Calories • 2.4g Carbs (0.7g Fiber) • 13.5g Fat • 58.3g Protein

Ingredients scaled to: 4 servings

- 3 cups Baby Spinach (85 grams)
- 1 3/4 cups Mushrooms sliced (168 grams)
- 3 stalks Green Onions (3 green onions, sliced) (36 grams)
- 1 tbsp Olive oil (13.5 grams)
- 4 Chicken breasts, bone and skin removed (944 grams)
- 1 dash Salt (0.40 grams)
- 1 dash Pepper (0.10 grams)
- 2 slices (1 oz) Provolone cheese (2 slices, halved) (56 grams)

Directions based on 4 servings

1. Preheat the grill to medium heat.
2. In a large skillet, sauté the spinach, mushrooms, and onions in oil until mushrooms are tender. Set aside and keep warm. Sprinkle chicken with salt and pepper.
3. Place chicken on a greased grill rack. Grill covered for about 4-5 minutes on each side or until a meat thermometer reads 165°F.

4. Top with cheese. Cover and grill 2-3 minutes longer or until the cheese is melted. Top chicken breasts with spinach and mushroom mixture. Enjoy!

BAKED CHICKEN WITH SPINACH, PEARS AND BLUE CHEESE

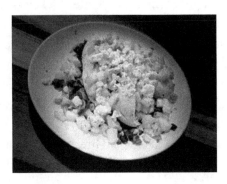

Per serving: 404 Calories • 21.4g Carbs (4.6g Fiber) • 20.8g Fat • 33.4g Protein

Ingredients scaled to: 4 Servings

- 2 Chicken breasts (filet) cut in half (472 grams)
- 3 tbsp Olive oil (40.5 grams)
- 1/2 cup chopped Red Onion (80 grams)
- 4 cups Spinach (120 grams)
- 2 tbsp Vinegar (29.8 grams)
- 2 large Pears skin removed (460 grams)
- 2 tbsp Parsley (7.6 grams)
- 3/4 cup crumbled Blue cheese (101 grams)

Directions based on 4 Servings

1. Preheat the oven to 375°F. With the chicken breast laying flat on a cutting surface, slowly cut horizontally through the thickest part to make 4 chicken breasts. Generously season each chicken breast with salt and pepper. In a large, oven-proof skillet, heat 1 tablespoon olive oil and sear breasts 2 to 3 minutes each side until lightly golden. Place the pan in the

oven and bake until chicken is cooked through, about 15 minutes.

2. Slice pears and put them aside. While chicken is cooking, heat 1 tablespoon of olive oil in a large pan over medium heat and sauté´ red onion until just softened, 2 to 3 minutes. Add spinach and toss until wilted. Season with salt and pepper and transfer to a large platter or divide evenly between 4 plates.

3. Wipe out the pan and heat the remaining 1 tablespoon olive oil with vinegar. Add pears and gently heat until warm. Stir in parsley. Arrange cooked chicken breasts on spinach. Top with warmed pear slices and about 2 tablespoons of blue cheese per breast.

LEMON GRILLED CHICKEN BREAST

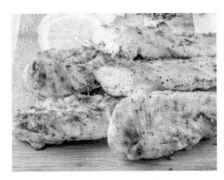

Per serving: 201 Calories • 0.81g Carbs • 10g Fat • 26g Protein

Ingredients scaled to: 4 servings

- 3 tbsp Lemon juice (45 grams)
- 2 tbsp Olive oil (27 grams)
- 2 cloves, minced Garlic (6 grams)
- 1 lb of Boneless Skinless Chicken breasts (454 grams)
- 1 dash Salt (0.40 grams)
- 1 dash Pepper (0.10 grams)
- Cooking spray (0.30 grams)

Directions based on 4 servings

1. Prepare the grill to medium-high heat. Combine the first 4 ingredients in a large zip-top plastic bag: seal. Marinate in the refrigerator for 30 minutes, turning occasionally. Remove chicken from bag, discard marinade. Sprinkle chicken evenly with salt and pepper.
2. Place chicken on a grill rack coated with cooking spray; grill 6 minutes on each side or until cooked through and no longer pink.
3. Enjoy!

GRILLED SALMON WITH DILL BUTTER

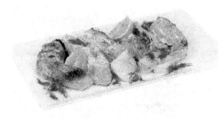

Per serving: 411 Calories • 2.9g Carbs (1.3g Fiber) • 29.4g Fat • 34.2g Protein

Ingredients scaled to: 4 servings

- 24 oz Atlantic salmon - with skin (680 grams)
- 2 tbsp Vegetable oil (28 grams)
- 1 Lemon Sliced (108 grams)
- 2 tsp Fresh Dill chopped (0.37 grams)
- 1/4 cup room temperature Butter (56.8 grams)
- 1 dash Salt (0.40 grams)

Directions based on 4 servings

1. Remove the salmon from the refrigerator and sprinkle it with a little salt. Let it sit at room temperature while you preheat your grill on high.
2. While the grill is heating, mix the fresh dill with the butter in a small bowl.
3. When the grill is hot, scrape down the grates with a grill brush. Pour a little vegetable oil onto a paper towel and use tongs to wipe down the grill grates. Coat the salmon in the remaining 2 tablespoons of oil and place, skin side up, onto the grill grates. Grill over high heat for 2-4 minutes,

depending on how thick your salmon pieces are. Carefully turn the salmon with a spatula. If using a gas grill, reduce the heat to medium. If using a charcoal grill, move the salmon to the cooler side of the grill. Cover and grill it for another 3-5 minutes, depending on how well done you prefer your salmon.

4. To serve, place a few thin slices of lemon on each plate. Remove the salmon pieces from the grill and place on the lemon slices. Top each piece of salmon with about a tablespoon of the dill butter and serve.

CHICKEN AND BROCCOLI

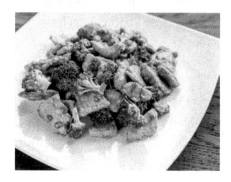

Per serving: 352 Calories • 7.2g Carbs (2.2g Fiber) • 10g Fat • 56.4g Protein

Ingredients scaled to: 4 servings

- 3 cups chopped Broccoli (273 grams)
- 1/2 cup, chopped Onions (80 grams)
- 1 tbsp Olive oil (13.5 grams)
- 4 Chicken breasts, bone and skin removed (944 grams)
- 1/2 cup Chicken broth (120 grams)
- 3 tbsp Soy sauce (48 grams)

Directions based on 4 servings

1. Chop broccoli. Bring water to boil in a pan with a steam tray. Place broccoli in a steam tray, cover, and steam for 4-6 minutes until broccoli has reached desired tenderness. Rinse under cold water and set aside.
2. In a 10" skillet or wok, heat the oil. Add the onion and cook until translucent. Add the broccoli and cook, stirring frequently, until onions begin to caramelize. Remove from the pan and return the pan to the heat.
3. Chop chicken. Add to the pan and cook until no longer pink. Return vegetables to the pan and mix together well.

4. Add in the chicken broth and soy sauce.
5. Eat hot and enjoy!

CHEESY CHICKEN AND SPINACH

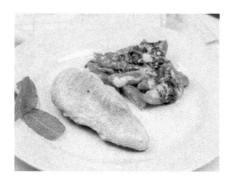

Per serving: 508 Calories • 7.7g Carbs (2.4g Fiber) • 24.7g Fat • 62.2g Protein

Ingredients scaled to: 1 serving

- 1 tbsp Olive oil (13.5 grams)
- 1 Chicken breast boneless and skinless (236 grams)
- 1 cup Spinach (30 grams)
- 1 cup Cherry tomatoes (149 grams)
- 1 oz Mozzarella cheese (28.4 grams)

Directions based on 1 serving

1. Heat olive oil in a skillet over medium-high heat. Add chicken, cooking for about 5-7 minutes. Flip chicken and continue to cook another 5-7 minutes until internal temperatures reach 165°F.
2. While the chicken is cooking, cut up tomatoes and spinach into bite-sized pieces.
3. Sauté vegetables in a separate pan, season with salt as desired.
4. Shred or grate mozzarella, and add to the pan.
5. When chicken is done cooking, remove it from heat. You can either smother the chicken or stuff it with the vegetable and cheese mixture.

BACON AND BRUSSELS SPROUTS GRATIN

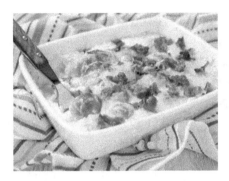

Per serving: 266 Calories • 6g Carbs (2.2g Fiber) • 23.2g Fat • 9.5g Protein

Ingredients scaled to: 8 servings

- 3 tbsp Butter (1 tbsp, cut into pieces) (28.4 grams)
- 8 oz Bacon (227 grams)
- 1 lb Brussels sprouts (Outer leaves and stems removed) (453 grams)
- 1/8 tsp Crushed red pepper flakes (0.040 grams)
- 1 dash Pepper (0.10 grams)
- 1 dash Salt (0.40 grams)
- 1/2 cup, Heavy whipping cream (119 grams)
- 1/2 cup, shredded Cheddar cheese (56.5 grams)

Directions based on 8 servings

1. Preheat the oven to 400°F.
2. Remove any brown outer leaves of brussel sprouts and trim stems. Set aside.
3. Use 2 tbsp of butter to grease a 2-quart baking dish.
4. Bring a large pot of water to a boil then add the salt. Add the Brussels sprouts and cook until tender, 8 to 10 minutes. Drain

the Brussels sprouts and coarsely chop. Fry bacon in a nonstick or cast iron pan until crisp and then coarsely chop.

5. Transfer sprouts and HALF of the bacon to the prepared baking dish and toss with the red pepper flakes, and salt and pepper to taste, then spread out evenly. Pour the cream on top and add the shredded cheese, crumbled bacon, and dot with the one tbsp of cut up butter.

6. Bake the gratin until bubbly and golden brown, about 15 minutes. Remove from the oven. Serve and enjoy!

BALSAMIC RED WINE GLAZED FILET MIGNON

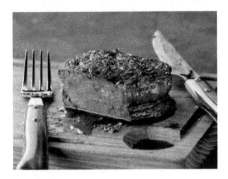

Per serving: 222 Calories • 6.5g Carbs (0.1g Fiber) • 6.7g Fat • 25.3g Protein

Ingredients scaled to: 2 servings

- 2 (4 oz) Beef tenderloins (227 grams)
- 1/2 tsp Pepper (1.1 grams)
- 1 tsp Salt (6 grams)
- 1/4 cup Balsamic vinegar (63.8 grams)
- 2 fl oz Red wine (58.8 grams)

Directions based on 2 servings

1. Sprinkle freshly ground pepper over both sides of each steak, and sprinkle with salt to taste.
2. Heat a nonstick skillet over medium-high heat. Place steaks in a hot pan, and cook for 1 minute on each side, or until browned. Reduce heat to medium-low and add balsamic vinegar and red wine. Cover, and cook for 4 minutes on each side, basting with sauce when you turn the meat over.
3. Remove steaks to two warmed plates, spoon one tablespoon of glaze over each, and serve immediately.

LEMON STEAMED BROCCOLI

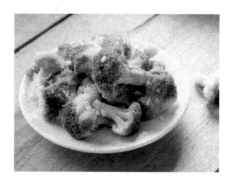

Per serving: 89 Calories • 11.7g Carbs (4.6g Fiber) • 4g Fat • 4.8g Protein

Ingredients scaled to: 4 servings

- 1 1/2 lbs **Broccoli** (680 grams)
- 1 tsp **Salt** (6 grams)
- 1 tsp **Pepper** (2.1 grams)
- 1 tbsp **Olive oil** (13.5 grams)
- 1/2 tsp **Lemon juice** (2.5 grams)

Directions based on 4 servings

1. Trim the broccoli into large florets.
2. Place the broccoli in a steaming basket over boiling water; cover and steam for 3 minutes.
3. Remove the lid for a moment, then cook, partially covered, until the stems are tender-firm, another 8-10 minutes.
4. Remove to a platter; season with salt and pepper, olive oil, and the lemon juice.
5. This recipe can be used as a side dish for many of the items listed above.

13
SNACK IDEAS

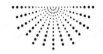

Everyone I know is looking for solace, hope, and a tasty snack. –Maira
Kalman

These snack ideas are best suited for the time-restricted methods of 16:8, 14:10, 12:12, and the longer fasting methods of 5/2, and Alternate Day Fasting.

ANTS ON A LOG

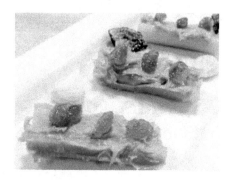

Per serving: 417 Calories • 43.3g Carbs (5.9g Fiber) • 25g Fat • 12.8g Protein

Ingredients scaled to: 1 serving

- 2 stalks, large (11 inches long) Celery (128 grams)
- 3 tbsp Peanut butter (48 grams)
- 1/4 cup Raisins (36.3 grams)

Directions based on 1 serving

1. Wash Celery, smear peanut butter into the inside of celery. Place raisins in peanut butter and enjoy!

APPLES AND ALMOND BUTTER

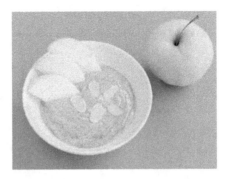

Per serving: 291 Calories • 31.1g Carbs (7.7g Fiber) • 18.1g Fat • 7.2g Protein

Ingredients scaled to: 1 apple

- 2 tbsp Almond butter (32 grams)
- 1 medium (3" dia) Apples (182 grams)

Directions based on 1 apple

1. Core and quarter a medium apple. Spread with almond butter and enjoy

CINNAMON APPLE BITES

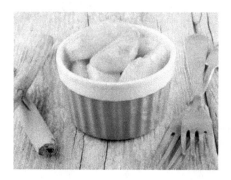

Per serving: 81 Calories • 21.6g Carbs (2.8g Fiber) • 0.2g Fat • 0.5g Protein

Ingredients scaled to: 1 serving

- 1 medium (3" dia) Apple (161 grams)
- 1/2 tsp Cinnamon (1.3 grams)

Directions based on 1 serving

1. Cut up the apple (with or without skin) into bite sized chunks.
2. Put the chopped apple into a container with a lid.
3. Sprinkle on the cinnamon, put the lid on the container, and gently shake so cinnamon covers the apple.
4. Eat and enjoy immediately.

APPLE AND VANILLA-CINNAMON YOGURT

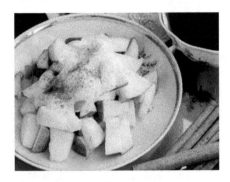

Per serving (one apple): 309 Calories • 61g Carbs (5.8g Fiber) • 3.4g Fat • 12.6g Protein

Ingredients scaled to: 1 apple

- 1 medium (3" dia) Apple (182 grams)
- 1 tsp Cinnamon (2.6 grams)
- 1 cup (8 fl oz) Vanilla yogurt (245 grams)

Directions based on 1 apple

1. Core and chop a medium apple. Mix into the yogurt and sprinkle with cinnamon. Enjoy!

PALEO & KETO CHOCOLATE PUDDING

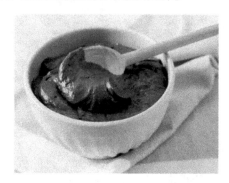

Per serving: 497 Calories • 17g Carbs (11.3g Fiber) • 49.1g Fat • 4.7g Protein

Ingredients scaled to: 2 servings

- 1/2 cup Coconut milk (120 grams)
- 2 Avocados, without skin and pit (272 grams)
- 1 tsp Vanilla extract (4.2 grams)
- 1 tsp Cocoa powder (1.8 grams)
- 2 dash Salt (0.80 grams)
- 4 tsp Coconut oil (18 grams)

Directions based on 2 serving

1. Add coconut milk, coconut oil and cocoa powder to a saucepan over medium heat. Heat up, whisking to combine, until the ingredients have incorporated. Remove from heat.
2. Stir in vanilla extract, and salt. Add avocado and blend using an immersion blender. Alternatively, transfer to a food processor and blend until smooth.
3. Enjoy at room temperature or chill.

BLUEBERRY MUFFIN

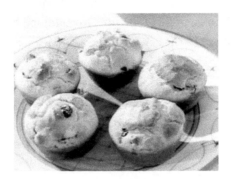

Per serving (one muffin): 171 Calories • 12.4g Carbs (3.9g Fiber) • 9.5g Fat • 11.3g Protein

Ingredients scaled to: 6 servings (6 muffins)

- Cooking spray (0.30 grams)
- 2 tbsp Wheat bran (7.3 grams)
- 1 cup Soy flour (105 grams)
- 1 tsp Baking powder (5 grams)
- 3 tsp Unrefined Cane Sugar (12 grams)
- 2 extra large Eggs room temperature (112 grams)
- 1/2 cups Heavy whipping cream (119 grams)
- 2 2/3 fl oz Club Soda (80 grams)
- 1/2 cup Blueberries (74 grams)

Directions based on 6 servings

1. Preheat the oven to 375°F.
2. Spray a 6-cup muffin tin with cooking spray. Evenly sprinkle the pan with the wheat bran and soy flour mix, being careful to coat the sides of the cups also; this will prevent sticking.
3. In a bowl using a wire whisk, mix all the remaining ingredients, except the blueberries, until well blended. Then

fold in the blueberries and fill the 6 muffin cups evenly with the batter. Place on the center rack of the oven and bake for 20 to 25 minutes, or until the tops turn golden brown and a toothpick stuck in the center comes out clean. Serve warm with butter or cold with cream cheese.

FROZEN YOGURT BLUEBERRIES

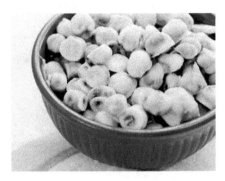

Per serving: Calories 175 Carbs 35g Fat 2g Protein 7g

Ingredients scaled to: 2 servings

- 1 tbsp Sugar (12.6 grams)
- 1 cup (8 fl oz) Vanilla yogurt (Greek or regular) (245 grams)
- 120 berries Blueberries (163 grams)

Directions based on 2 servings

1. 1Line a baking sheet with parchment and set aside.
2. In a medium bowl, mix the sugar and yogurt together.
3. Gently fold in blueberries to coat in the yogurt. Scoop them up with a fork and tap off excess.
4. Place the blueberries on the baking sheet, being careful not to have them touch.
5. Freeze the baking sheet until the blueberries are completely frozen, about 1 hour.
6. Store leftovers in an airtight container in the freezer.

MANGO SMOOTHIE

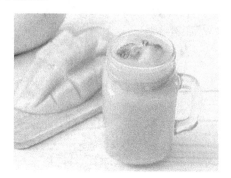

Per serving: 170 Calories • 39.9g Carbs (6g Fiber) • 1.2g Fat • 3.4g Protein

Ingredients scaled to: 2 servings (2 smoothies)

- 2 Mangos, without skin and pit (414 grams)
- 2 cups Coconut water (liquid from coconuts) (480 grams)
- 2 cups Ice cubes (474 grams)

Directions

1. Combine all ingredients in a blender and pulse until smooth. Enjoy!

GREEK YOGURT WITH BLUEBERRIES, WALNUTS & HONEY

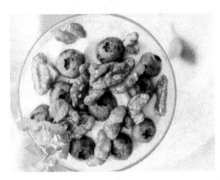

Per serving: 405 Calories • 18.4g Carbs (3g Fiber) • 30.6g Fat • 17.7g Protein

Ingredients scaled to: 1 serving

- 1/4 cup Blueberries (37 grams)
- 1 tsp Honey (7.1 grams)
- 1/4 cup chopped Walnuts (31.3 grams)
- 1/2 cup Greek yogurt (120 grams)

Directions based on 1 serving

1. Mix the ingredients together and enjoy!

RICE CAKE WITH STRAWBERRIES AND HONEY

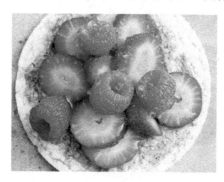

Per serving: 125 Calories • 31g Carbs (2.1g Fiber) • 0.5g Fat • 1.4g Protein

Ingredients scaled to: 1 serving

- ½ cup, sliced Strawberries (83 grams)
- 1 tbsp Honey (21 grams)
- 1 Rice cake (9 grams)

Directions based on 1 serving

1. Slice strawberries. Place on rice cake and drizzle with honey. Enjoy!

SPINACH AVOCADO SMOOTHIE BOWL

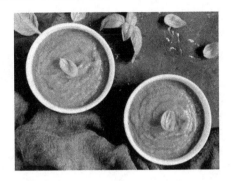

Per serving: 154 Calories • 7.3g Carbs (5.1g Fiber) • 13.2g Fat • 1.9g Protein

Ingredients scaled to: 1 serving

- 2 cups Baby Spinach (56.7 grams)
- 1/2 Avocado - without skin and pit (68 grams)
- 2/3 cup (8 fl oz) Unsweetened Coconut Milk (160 grams)

Directions based on 1 serving

1. Blend and serve with any desired toppings. Enjoy!

14
21-DAY MEAL PLAN

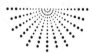

You are what you eat so don't be fast, cheap, easy, or fake. –Unknown

The 16:8 IF method is the most popular and commonplace for people to start theirs IF journey. Therefore, the meal plan outlined in this chapter will be based on the 16:8 IF method utilizing meals found in the recipe chapters.

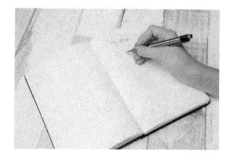

SAMPLE MEAL PLAN FOR 16:8

WEEK 1

Monday

- Breakfast: Scrambled Eggs with Spinach and Cheese
- Lunch: BBQ Chicken Salad
- Snack: Ants on a Log
- Dinner: Grilled Salmon with Dill Butter

Tuesday

- Breakfast: Protein Berry and Carrot Smoothie
- Lunch: Turkey Salad
- Snack: Ants on a Log
- Dinner: Maple Glazed Chicken

Wednesday

- Breakfast: Cottage Cheese & Applesauce
- Lunch: Chicken Lettuce Wraps
- Snack: Apples and Almond Butter
- Dinner: Peppered Steaks with Mushrooms

Thursday

- Breakfast: Strawberry Yogurt Smoothie
- Lunch: Spinach, Lemon, and Shrimp Salad
- Snack: Cinnamon Apple Bites
- Dinner: Philly Cheesesteak Stuffed Peppers

Friday

- Breakfast: Scrambled Eggs with Spinach and Cheese

- Lunch: Chicken, Spinach, and Strawberry Salad
- Snack: Spinach Avocado Smoothie Bowl
- Dinner: Spinach and Mushroom Smothered Grilled Chicken

Saturday

- Breakfast: Keto Breakfast Tacos
- Lunch: BBQ Chicken Salad
- Snack: Paleo & Keto Chocolate Pudding
- Dinner: Grilled Salmon with Dill Butter

Sunday

- Breakfast: Spinach and Sausage Breakfast Muffins
- Lunch: Cheesy Burger Stuffed Portobellos
- Snack: Blueberry Muffin
- Dinner: Chicken and Broccoli

WEEK 2

Monday

- Breakfast: Kale and Egg Cups
- Lunch: Paleo Avocado Chicken Salad
- Snack: Frozen Yogurt Blueberries
- Dinner: Cheesy Chicken and Spinach

Tuesday

- Breakfast: Oatmeal and Apples
- Lunch: Paleo Avocado Tuna Salad
- Snack: Rice Cake with Strawberries and Honey
- Dinner: Bacon and Brussels Sprouts Gratin

Wednesday

- Breakfast: Soft Boiled Eggs & Toast
- Lunch: Mexican Quinoa
- Snack: Ants on a Log
- Dinner: Balsamic Red Wine Glazed Filet Mignon

Thursday

- Breakfast: Peanut Butter Banana English Muffin
- Lunch: BBQ Chicken Salad
- Snack: Paleo & Keto Chocolate Pudding
- Dinner: Baked Chicken with Spinach, Pears and Blue Cheese

Friday

- Breakfast: Kale and Egg Cup
- Lunch: Chicken Lettuce Wraps
- Snack: Mango Smoothie
- Dinner: Philly Cheesesteak Stuffed Peppers

Saturday

- Breakfast: Strawberry Yogurt Smoothie
- Lunch: Spinach, Lemon, and Shrimp Salad
- Snack: Apples and Almond Butter
- Dinner: Peppered Steaks with Mushrooms

Sunday

- Breakfast: Keto Breakfast Tacos
- Lunch: Cheesy Burger Stuffed Portobellos
- Snack: Ants on a Log
- Dinner: Lemon Grilled Chicken Breast

WEEK 3

Monday

- Breakfast: Oatmeal and Apples
- Lunch: Turkey Salad
- Snack: Frozen Yogurt Blueberries
- Dinner: Maple Glazed Chicken

Tuesday

- Breakfast: Spinach and Sausage Breakfast Muffins
- Lunch: Flank Steak and Tomatoes
- Snack: Blueberry Muffin
- Dinner: Bacon and Brussels Sprouts Gratin

Wednesday

- Breakfast: Keto Breakfast Tacos
- Lunch: Paleo Avocado Tuna Salad
- Snack: Cinnamon Apple Bites
- Dinner: Baked Chicken with Spinach, Pears and Blue Cheese

Thursday

- Breakfast: Oatmeal and Apples
- Lunch: Mexican Quinoa
- Snack: Mango Smoothie
- Dinner: Chicken and Broccoli

Friday

- Breakfast: Peanut Butter Banana English Muffin

- Lunch: Chicken, Spinach, and Strawberry Salad
- Snack: Spinach Avocado Smoothie Bowl
- Dinner: Spinach and Mushroom Smothered Grilled Chicken

Saturday

- Breakfast: Kale and Egg Cups
- Lunch: Cheesy Burger Stuffed Portobellos
- Snack: Cinnamon Apple Bites
- Dinner: Balsamic Red Wine Glazed Filet Mignon

Sunday

- Breakfast: Strawberry Yogurt Smoothie
- Lunch: Spinach, Lemon, and Shrimp Salad
- Snack: Rice Cake with Strawberries and Honey
- Dinner: Philly Cheesesteak Stuffed Peppers

MEAL PLAN TEMPLATE

Monday

Breakfast:

Snack:

Lunch:

Dinner:

Tuesday

Breakfast:

Snack:

Lunch:

Dinner:

Wednesday

Breakfast:

Snack:

Lunch:

Dinner:

Thursday

Breakfast:

Snack:

Lunch:

Dinner:

Friday

Breakfast:

Snack:

Lunch:

Dinner:

Saturday

Breakfast:

Snack:

Lunch:

Dinner:

Sunday

Breakfast:

Snack:

Lunch:

Dinner:

PLEASE LEAVE A REVIEW

If you have found this book to be of value so far, please take a moment right now and leave an honest review of this book

This will take you less than a minute of your time. All you have to do is to leave a review.

Please go to the page on Amazon (or where you purchased this book) and leave a review.

Thank you for your kindness.

CPSIA information can be obtained
at www.ICGtesting.com
Printed in the USA
LVHW050148160723
752292LV00008B/1089